OWEN HUNTER

Eczema

Your Comprehensive Blueprint for Diagnosis and Treatment

Copyright © 2024 by Owen Hunter

All rights reserved. No part of this publication may be reproduced, stored or transmitted in any form or by any means, electronic, mechanical, photocopying, recording, scanning, or otherwise without written permission from the publisher. It is illegal to copy this book, post it to a website, or distribute it by any other means without permission.

First edition

This book was professionally typeset on Reedsy.
Find out more at reedsy.com

Contents

INTRODUCTION

Unveiling the Mystery of Eczema

Imagine waking up every morning, your skin itching and burning, red patches scattered across your body like an unwelcome map of discomfort. For millions of people worldwide, this isn't just imagination—it's their daily reality. Eczema, a term that encompasses a group of inflammatory skin conditions, affects an estimated 10% of the global population. It's more than just a skin problem; it's a complex, often misunderstood condition that can significantly impact quality of life, mental health, and overall well-being.

If you're holding this book, chances are you're familiar with the frustration, discomfort, and sometimes even despair that comes with eczema. Perhaps you're a long-time sufferer, searching for new insights and strategies to manage your condition. Maybe you're a parent, watching helplessly as your child struggles with itchy, inflamed skin. Or you could be a healthcare professional, seeking to deepen your understanding of this pervasive condition. Whoever you are, whatever your relationship with eczema, you've come to the right place.

"Mastering Eczema: A Comprehensive Guide to Understanding, Managing, and Thriving with Skin Inflammation" is not just another book about skin conditions. It's a journey—a deep dive into the world of eczema, exploring its causes, manifestations, and management from every angle. Our goal is to empower you with knowledge, equip you with practical strategies, and inspire hope in your journey towards healthier skin and a better quality of life.

The Eczema Epidemic

Eczema, particularly atopic dermatitis—its most common form—has been on the rise in recent decades. This increase is particularly pronounced in industrialized countries, leading some researchers to dub it an "epidemic of an allergic disease." But why? What factors in our modern world are contributing to this surge in inflammatory skin conditions?

The answers, as we'll explore throughout this book, are multifaceted and sometimes surprising. From changes in our diet and lifestyle to shifts in our environment and even our obsession with cleanliness (the so-called "hygiene hypothesis"), numerous factors seem to be at play. Understanding these underlying causes is crucial not just for managing eczema, but for potentially preventing its onset or reducing its severity.

Beyond the Itch: The True Impact of Eczema

When we think of eczema, the first things that often come to mind are its visible symptoms: red, inflamed skin; dry, scaly patches; and sometimes oozing or crusting. But the impact of eczema goes far beyond skin-deep. The persistent itch can disrupt sleep, leading to fatigue, irritability, and decreased productivity. The visible nature of the condition can affect self-esteem and social interactions, sometimes leading to anxiety and depression.

For children with eczema, the effects can be particularly profound. Studies have shown that children with moderate to severe eczema are more likely to struggle in school, both academically and socially. They may avoid activities like swimming or sports due to embarrassment or discomfort, potentially impacting their physical health and social development.

Even for adults, eczema can have far-reaching consequences. It can affect career choices, romantic relationships, and overall quality of life. The financial burden of managing eczema—from doctor's visits and prescription medications to special skincare products and clothing—can also be significant.

By understanding these wider impacts, we can approach eczema management more holistically, addressing not just the physical symptoms but also the emotional and social aspects of living with a chronic skin condition.

The Science of Skin: Understanding Eczema from the Inside Out

To truly understand eczema, we need to start at the cellular level. Our skin is an incredible organ—the largest in the human body. It serves as a barrier, protecting us from environmental threats, regulating our body temperature, and even synthesizing vital nutrients like Vitamin D.

In people with eczema, this skin barrier is compromised. The exact mechanisms can vary depending on the type of eczema, but generally, there's a combination of genetic predisposition and environmental factors at play. Some people with eczema lack sufficient filaggrin, a protein crucial for maintaining the skin barrier. Others may have an overactive immune response, causing inflammation even in response to harmless substances.

Throughout this book, we'll delve deeper into the science behind eczema. We'll explore the role of the immune system, the impact of the skin microbiome, and the latest research on genetic factors. By understanding these underlying mechanisms, we can better appreciate why certain treatments work and how lifestyle changes can make a significant difference.

Breaking Down Barriers: Dispelling Eczema Myths

Despite its prevalence, eczema remains shrouded in misconceptions. "It's just dry skin," some might say. Or, "You'll grow out of it eventually." Perhaps you've heard that eczema is contagious, or that it's caused by poor hygiene. These myths not only contribute to the stigma surrounding eczema but can also lead to ineffective or even harmful management strategies.

In this book, we'll tackle these myths head-on, replacing them with evidence-based information. We'll explore questions like: Can diet really impact eczema? Is eczema always a lifelong condition? How does stress affect skin inflammation? By addressing these common misconceptions, we aim to provide a clearer, more accurate picture of what eczema is—and isn't.

A Holistic Approach to Eczema Management

When it comes to managing eczema, there's no one-size-fits-all solution. What works for one person may be ineffective or even problematic for another. That's why this book advocates for a holistic, personalized approach to eczema care.

We'll explore a wide range of management strategies, from conventional medical treatments to alternative therapies. We'll discuss the latest in prescription medications, including topical corticosteroids, immunomodulators, and biologic drugs. But we'll also delve into natural remedies, dietary approaches, and lifestyle modifications that can complement medical treatments.

Importantly, we'll emphasize the need for an individualized approach. Eczema can manifest differently from person to person, and its triggers can be highly individual. By understanding your unique eczema profile—your triggers, your symptoms, your response to different treatments—you can develop a management plan that works best for you.

The Emotional Journey: Coping with a Chronic Condition

Living with eczema isn't just a physical challenge—it's an emotional one too.

The unpredictable nature of flare-ups can lead to feelings of frustration and helplessness. The visible nature of the condition can impact self-esteem and social confidence. And the constant vigilance required—avoiding triggers, sticking to skincare routines, managing stress—can be mentally exhausting.

Throughout this book, we'll address the psychological aspects of living with eczema. We'll explore coping strategies, discuss the importance of self-care, and provide tips for building resilience. We'll also look at the role of stress in eczema flare-ups and explore techniques for stress management that can benefit both your skin and your overall well-being.

For parents of children with eczema, we'll offer guidance on supporting your child emotionally as well as physically. We'll discuss how to build your child's self-esteem, manage school and social situations, and gradually transfer responsibility for eczema management as your child grows older.

The Power of Community: You're Not Alone

One of the most challenging aspects of living with eczema can be the feeling of isolation. You might feel like no one understands what you're going through, or that you're alone in your struggles. But the truth is, millions of people around the world are on similar journeys.

In this book, we'll highlight the importance of community in managing eczema. We'll explore the benefits of support groups, both in-person and online, and provide resources for connecting with others who understand your experiences. We'll also discuss the role of patient advocacy organizations in providing support, driving research, and influencing healthcare policies.

By sharing stories from real people living with eczema, we hope to remind you that you're not alone in this journey. These personal accounts will offer not just comfort, but also practical tips and inspiration for managing your own eczema.

Looking to the Future: Hope on the Horizon

While living with eczema can be challenging, there's reason for optimism. Research into the causes and treatment of eczema is advancing rapidly. New therapies are being developed, our understanding of the condition is deepening, and management strategies are becoming more sophisticated and personalized.

In the final chapters of this book, we'll look towards the future of eczema care. We'll explore emerging treatments, including promising new biologics and potential gene therapies. We'll discuss advances in our understanding of the skin microbiome and how this might lead to novel treatment approaches. And we'll look at how technologies like artificial intelligence and telemedicine might transform eczema management in the coming years.

Your Eczema Journey Starts Here

As we embark on this exploration of eczema together, remember that knowledge is power. The more you understand about your condition, the better equipped you'll be to manage it effectively. But knowledge alone isn't enough—it's what you do with that knowledge that truly matters.

This book is designed to be more than just an informational resource. It's a tool for empowerment, a guide for action, and a source of hope. As you read, we encourage you to take notes, ask questions, and think about how you can apply what you're learning to your own life or the life of someone you care for.

Remember, managing eczema is a journey, not a destination. There may be setbacks along the way, but there will also be progress and moments of relief. By arming yourself with knowledge, developing a personalized management plan, and connecting with a supportive community, you can take control of your eczema rather than letting it control you.

So, let's begin this journey together. Whether you're newly diagnosed or have been living with eczema for years, whether you're struggling with severe symptoms or looking to maintain periods of remission, this book is for you. Turn the page, and let's start unraveling the mystery of eczema, one chapter at a time.

CHAPTER 1

Understanding Eczema: The Basics

Eczema, a term that often evokes images of red, itchy skin, is far more complex and multifaceted than many people realize. In this chapter, we'll lay the groundwork for understanding this common yet often misunderstood condition. We'll explore what eczema is, the various types that exist, and just how prevalent this condition is in our modern world.

What is Eczema?

At its core, eczema is a group of inflammatory skin conditions characterized by itchy, inflamed skin. The word "eczema" itself comes from the Greek word "ekzein," which means "to boil out" or "to effervesce." This vivid description aptly captures the appearance of eczematous skin during flare-ups.

Eczema is not a single condition but rather an umbrella term encompassing several related skin disorders. These conditions share common symptoms but can have different causes, triggers, and patterns of occurrence. The most common form of eczema is atopic dermatitis, but as we'll explore later in this chapter, there are several other types as well.

Key Characteristics of Eczema

While the specific manifestations of eczema can vary from person to person and between different types of the condition, there are several hallmark characteristics:

1. Itching (Pruritus): This is often the most distressing symptom of eczema. The itch can be intense and persistent, leading to a vicious cycle of scratching and further skin damage.

2. Inflammation: Eczematous skin is typically red and swollen due to the inflammatory response occurring in the skin.

3. Dryness: The skin often appears dry, rough, and may have a scaly texture.

4. Skin Barrier Dysfunction: People with eczema have a compromised skin barrier, making their skin more susceptible to irritants, allergens, and moisture loss.

5. Recurring Nature: Eczema is typically characterized by periods of flare-ups followed by periods of remission.

6. Location Specificity: Different types of eczema tend to affect specific areas of the body, which can aid in diagnosis.

The Eczema Cycle

Understanding the cyclical nature of eczema is crucial for effective management. The typical eczema cycle involves:

1. Trigger Exposure: This could be contact with an irritant, an allergic reaction, stress, or other factors we'll explore in later chapters.

2. Inflammation: The immune system responds to the trigger, leading to inflammation in the skin.

3. Itching: The inflammation causes intense itching.

4. Scratching: The natural response to itching is to scratch, which can damage the skin further.

5. Skin Barrier Damage: Scratching compromises the skin barrier, making it more susceptible to irritants and moisture loss.

6. Increased Vulnerability: The damaged skin barrier allows for easier entry of irritants and allergens, potentially leading to more inflammation.

7. Cycle Repeats: Without intervention, this cycle can continue, leading to chronic inflammation and skin damage.

Breaking this cycle is a key goal in eczema management, which we'll discuss in detail in later chapters.

Types of Eczema

While atopic dermatitis is the most common and well-known form of eczema, there are several other types. Understanding these different forms is crucial for proper diagnosis and treatment. Let's explore each type in detail:

1. Atopic Dermatitis

Atopic dermatitis is the most common form of eczema, affecting up to 20% of children and 3% of adults worldwide. It's a chronic condition that often begins in childhood and may persist into adulthood.

Key features of atopic dermatitis include:
   - Typically begins in infancy or early childhood
   - Often associated with other atopic conditions like asthma and hay fever
   - Tends to affect specific areas of the body, such as the face, hands, feet,

and flexural areas (inside of elbows and knees)
   - Can have a significant impact on quality of life due to intense itching and visible skin changes

2. Contact Dermatitis

Contact dermatitis occurs when the skin comes into contact with a substance that either irritates it or triggers an allergic reaction. There are two main types:

a) Irritant Contact Dermatitis: This is the most common type, occurring when the skin is exposed to a substance that physically, chemically, or mechanically damages the skin. Common irritants include soaps, detergents, and certain workplace chemicals.

b) Allergic Contact Dermatitis: This occurs when the skin comes into contact with a substance to which the individual has developed an allergy. Common allergens include nickel, fragrances, and certain plants like poison ivy.

3. Seborrheic Dermatitis

Seborrheic dermatitis affects areas of the body with a high concentration of sebaceous (oil-producing) glands. It's characterized by red, scaly patches and can affect the scalp (where it's often known as dandruff), face, upper chest, and back.

Key features include:
   - Often affects the scalp, eyebrows, sides of the nose, and behind the ears
   - Can be exacerbated by stress or changes in humidity
   - May be related to an overgrowth of a yeast that naturally lives on the skin

4. Dyshidrotic Eczema

Also known as pompholyx, dyshidrotic eczema is characterized by small, intensely itchy blisters on the edges of the fingers, toes, palms, and soles of the feet.

Key features include:
  - More common in women than men
  - Often triggered by stress, allergies, or exposure to certain metals (like nickel)
  - Can be associated with hyperhidrosis (excessive sweating)

5. Nummular Eczema

Nummular eczema, also called discoid eczema, is characterized by circular or oval patches of irritated skin. The word "nummular" comes from the Latin word for "coin," reflecting the round shape of the lesions.

Key features include:
  - Can occur at any age but is more common in older adults
  - Often appears after a skin injury, such as a burn, insect bite, or abrasion
  - Lesions can be very itchy and may ooze fluid

6. Stasis Dermatitis

Stasis dermatitis occurs when there's poor circulation in the lower legs, typically due to varicose veins or other conditions that affect blood flow. This leads to fluid build-up and skin inflammation.

Key features include:
  - Most common in older adults
  - Typically affects the lower legs
  - May be accompanied by leg swelling, varicose veins, and skin discoloration

7. Neurodermatitis

Also known as lichen simplex chronicus, neurodermatitis is characterized by thick, scaly patches of skin caused by excessive scratching and rubbing.

Key features include:
   - Often begins with a patch of itchy skin
   - Constant scratching leads to thickened, leathery skin
   - Can be triggered by stress or other eczema types

Understanding these different types of eczema is crucial for several reasons. First, it helps in getting an accurate diagnosis. The treatment approach can vary depending on the type of eczema, so correct identification is key to effective management. Additionally, recognizing the specific type can provide insights into potential triggers and help in developing targeted prevention strategies.

Prevalence and Statistics

Eczema is a global health concern, affecting millions of people worldwide. Let's look at some key statistics to understand the scope of this condition:

Global Prevalence:
   - It's estimated that 15-20% of children and 1-3% of adults worldwide are affected by atopic dermatitis, the most common form of eczema.
   - The prevalence of eczema has increased two to three-fold in industrialized countries over the past few decades.

Regional Variations:
   - Eczema prevalence varies significantly between countries and even between regions within countries.
   - Generally, prevalence is higher in developed countries and urban areas compared to rural areas.

Age Distribution:
 - Eczema often begins in childhood, with up to 20% of children affected.
 - While many children outgrow eczema, about 50% continue to have symptoms into adulthood.
 - Adult-onset eczema, while less common, affects about 1 in 4 adults with eczema.

Gender Differences:
 - In childhood, eczema affects boys and girls roughly equally.
 - In adulthood, eczema is slightly more common in women than in men.

Economic Impact:
 - The economic burden of eczema is substantial, including direct medical costs and indirect costs such as lost productivity.
 - In the United States alone, the annual cost of eczema is estimated to be over $5 billion.

Quality of Life Impact:
 - Eczema can significantly impact quality of life, affecting sleep, work productivity, and social interactions.
 - Studies have shown that the quality of life impact of moderate to severe eczema is comparable to that of other chronic diseases like diabetes and heart disease.

Comorbidities:
 - People with eczema, particularly atopic dermatitis, are at increased risk for other health conditions.
 - These include other atopic conditions (asthma, hay fever), skin infections, and mental health issues like anxiety and depression.

These statistics highlight the widespread nature of eczema and its significant impact on individuals and society as a whole. They underscore the importance of continued research, improved management strategies, and increased public awareness about this condition.

The Rise of Eczema: Theories and Hypotheses

The increasing prevalence of eczema, particularly in developed countries, has led researchers to propose several theories about why this condition is on the rise. While the exact reasons are still being studied, several hypotheses have gained attention:

1. The Hygiene Hypothesis: This theory suggests that our increasingly clean environments may be reducing our exposure to beneficial microbes, leading to an overreactive immune system. This could explain why eczema is more common in urban, developed areas.

2. Environmental Factors: Increased exposure to pollutants, changes in diet, and the use of certain personal care products may be contributing to the rise in eczema cases.

3. Genetic Factors: While genetics alone don't explain the increase in prevalence, they play a crucial role in eczema susceptibility. As our understanding of genetics improves, we're discovering more about how genetic variations can influence eczema risk.

4. The Skin Microbiome: Recent research has highlighted the importance of the skin's microbiome (the community of microorganisms living on our skin) in skin health. Disruptions to this microbiome may contribute to eczema development.

5. Climate Change: Some researchers propose that climate change, leading to longer pollen seasons and changes in temperature and humidity, may be contributing to increased eczema prevalence.

These theories are not mutually exclusive, and it's likely that a combination of factors is responsible for the increasing prevalence of eczema. Ongoing research continues to shed light on this complex issue.

Conclusion: The Complexity of Eczema

As we've explored in this chapter, eczema is far more than just a simple skin condition. It's a complex, multifaceted disorder that can manifest in various forms and affect people of all ages. Understanding the basics of eczema—its definition, types, and prevalence—lays the foundation for deeper exploration of its causes, triggers, and management strategies.

The statistics we've discussed highlight the significant impact of eczema on individuals and society as a whole. They underscore the importance of continued research, improved treatments, and increased public awareness about this condition.

As we move forward in this book, we'll delve deeper into the science behind eczema, exploring its causes and triggers in detail. We'll examine the latest research and treatment options, and provide practical strategies for managing eczema in daily life. Whether you're dealing with eczema yourself, caring for someone with the condition, or simply seeking to understand it better, the knowledge we'll explore in the coming chapters will equip you to face the challenges of eczema with confidence and hope.

Remember, while eczema can be a challenging condition to live with, understanding it is the first step towards effective management. With the right knowledge and tools, it's possible to gain control over eczema and improve quality of life. As we continue our journey through this book, we'll equip you with the information and strategies you need to do just that.

CHAPTER 2

The Science Behind Eczema

Understanding the science behind eczema is crucial for effectively managing the condition. In this chapter, we'll delve into the intricate workings of the skin, explore how the immune system plays a role in eczema, and examine the genetic factors that contribute to its development. By the end of this chapter, you'll have a comprehensive understanding of the biological mechanisms underlying eczema.

The Skin: Our Body's First Line of Defense

To understand eczema, we must first understand the skin itself. The skin is our largest organ, covering an average of 20 square feet in adults. It serves as a protective barrier, regulating body temperature, preventing water loss, and defending against pathogens and environmental stressors.

The skin is composed of three main layers:

1. Epidermis: The outermost layer of the skin
2. Dermis: The layer beneath the epidermis, containing blood vessels, nerve endings, and hair follicles
3. Hypodermis: The deepest layer, primarily composed of fat cells

For our discussion of eczema, we'll focus primarily on the epidermis, as this is where most of the action related to eczema occurs.

The Epidermis: A Closer Look

The epidermis is made up of several layers of cells, primarily keratinocytes. These cells are produced in the deepest layer of the epidermis (the stratum basale) and gradually move upward, changing shape and composition until they reach the surface of the skin. This process, known as keratinization, takes about 28 days in healthy skin.

The uppermost layer of the epidermis, called the stratum corneum, is crucial for skin barrier function. It's often described as a "brick and mortar" structure:

- The "bricks" are corneocytes, which are flattened, dead keratinocytes filled with keratin proteins.
  - The "mortar" is a complex mixture of lipids, including ceramides, cholesterol, and free fatty acids.

This structure creates a waterproof barrier that prevents excessive water loss and keeps out harmful substances and microorganisms.

Skin Barrier Dysfunction in Eczema

In people with eczema, particularly atopic dermatitis, this skin barrier is compromised. Several factors contribute to this:

1. Filaggrin Deficiency: Filaggrin is a protein that plays a crucial role in the formation and hydration of the stratum corneum. Many people with eczema have mutations in the gene that codes for filaggrin, leading to a deficiency of this important protein.

2. Lipid Abnormalities: The composition and organization of lipids in the stratum corneum are often abnormal in eczematous skin, compromising its barrier function.

3. pH Imbalance: Healthy skin has a slightly acidic pH, which is important for antimicrobial defense and optimal function of skin enzymes. In eczema, the skin's pH is often higher (more alkaline), disrupting these processes.

4. Increased Trans-Epidermal Water Loss (TEWL): Due to the compromised barrier, water escapes more easily from the skin, leading to dryness and increased susceptibility to irritants.

This impaired skin barrier not only allows irritants and allergens to penetrate more easily but also triggers an immune response, leading to inflammation - a hallmark of eczema.

The Immune System: Friend or Foe?

The immune system plays a central role in eczema, particularly in atopic dermatitis. In healthy individuals, the immune system protects the body from harmful invaders like bacteria and viruses. However, in people with eczema, the immune system can overreact, leading to inflammation even in the absence of a true threat.

Key Players in the Immune Response

Several components of the immune system are involved in the development of eczema:

1. T Cells: These are a type of white blood cell that play a central role in cell-mediated immunity. In eczema, there's often an imbalance in T cell populations, with an increase in Th2 cells that promote inflammation.

2. Cytokines: These are small proteins released by cells that have a specific effect on the interactions and communications between cells. In eczema, there's often an overproduction of pro-inflammatory cytokines, particularly those associated with Th2 responses (like IL-4, IL-5, and IL-13).

3. Immunoglobulin E (IgE): Many people with atopic dermatitis have elevated levels of IgE, an antibody associated with allergic responses.

4. Langerhans Cells: These are immune cells found in the epidermis that play a role in triggering immune responses. In eczema, these cells may be more easily activated by environmental triggers.

The Atopic March

The concept of the "atopic march" is important in understanding the relationship between eczema and other allergic conditions. This term describes the typical progression of atopic diseases:

1. Eczema often appears first, usually in infancy or early childhood.
2. Food allergies may develop next, often in early childhood.
3. Asthma often follows, typically appearing in later childhood.
4. Allergic rhinitis (hay fever) often develops last, usually in the teenage years or early adulthood.

Not everyone with eczema will experience all of these conditions, but there's a strong association between them. This progression highlights the systemic nature of atopic conditions and the central role of the immune system in their development.

The Itch-Scratch Cycle

One of the most distressing aspects of eczema is the intense itch, medically termed pruritus. The itch-scratch cycle is a key feature of eczema that involves both the skin and the nervous system:

1. Inflammation in the skin activates nerve fibers that signal itch.
2. Scratching temporarily relieves the itch by providing a competing sensation.
3. However, scratching damages the skin, releasing more inflammatory mediators.
4. This leads to more inflammation and more itching, perpetuating the cycle.

Breaking this cycle is a key goal in eczema management, which we'll discuss in later chapters.

Genetic Factors in Eczema

Genetics plays a significant role in the development of eczema, particularly atopic dermatitis. While eczema isn't a simple genetic disorder - environmental factors also play a crucial role - there's strong evidence for a genetic component:

1. Family History: Children with one parent with atopic dermatitis have a 2-3 times higher risk of developing the condition. If both parents are affected, the risk is even higher.

2. Twin Studies: Identical twins are more likely to both have eczema compared to fraternal twins, indicating a genetic component.

3. Specific Gene Mutations: Several genes have been associated with increased eczema risk:

a) FLG Gene: As mentioned earlier, mutations in the filaggrin gene are strongly associated with atopic dermatitis. These mutations are found in up to 50% of people with moderate to severe atopic dermatitis.

b) SPINK5 Gene: This gene codes for a protein that helps regulate the shedding of skin cells. Mutations in this gene are associated with a rare form of eczema called Netherton syndrome.

c) Immune System Genes: Various genes involved in immune system function have been linked to eczema risk, including genes in the interleukin family (like IL-4 and IL-13) and genes involved in the regulation of IgE production.

It's important to note that having these genetic variations doesn't guarantee that a person will develop eczema. Environmental factors and gene-environment interactions also play crucial roles.

Epigenetics: Where Genes Meet Environment

The field of epigenetics - the study of how behaviors and environment can cause changes that affect the way genes work - is providing new insights into eczema. Epigenetic changes don't alter the DNA sequence but can change how the body reads a DNA sequence.

Several environmental factors have been shown to induce epigenetic changes that may influence eczema risk:

1. Diet: Maternal diet during pregnancy and early childhood diet may influence eczema risk through epigenetic mechanisms.

2. Stress: Both maternal stress during pregnancy and childhood stress have been associated with epigenetic changes that may increase eczema risk.

3. Pollution: Exposure to air pollution has been linked to epigenetic changes

that may increase susceptibility to eczema.

4. Microbiome: The community of microorganisms living on and in our bodies can influence gene expression through epigenetic mechanisms.

Understanding these epigenetic factors opens up new possibilities for eczema prevention and treatment, which researchers are actively exploring.

The Skin Microbiome: A New Frontier

In recent years, there's been growing interest in the role of the skin microbiome in eczema. The skin microbiome refers to the community of microorganisms - bacteria, fungi, and viruses - that live on our skin.

In healthy skin, these microorganisms live in a delicate balance, helping to protect against pathogens and maintain skin health. However, in eczema, this balance is often disrupted:

1. Reduced Diversity: People with eczema often have less diverse skin microbiomes compared to those without the condition.

2. Staphylococcus aureus: This bacteria is often found in higher numbers on eczematous skin, and its presence is associated with more severe symptoms.

3. Beneficial Bacteria: Some bacteria, like certain strains of Staphylococcus epidermidis, may help protect against eczema, but are often found in lower numbers in people with the condition.

Research into the skin microbiome is opening up new avenues for eczema treatment, including the development of "good" bacteria that could be applied to the skin to restore a healthy balance.

Inflammation: The Common Thread

Inflammation is a common thread running through all aspects of eczema - from the compromised skin barrier to the overactive immune response. Understanding the inflammatory process in eczema is crucial for developing effective treatments:

1. Acute Inflammation: This is the body's initial response to harmful stimuli. In eczema, this can be triggered by allergens, irritants, or even stress. Acute inflammation leads to the classic signs of eczema: redness, swelling, and itching.

2. Chronic Inflammation: If the inflammatory response persists, it becomes chronic. This can lead to ongoing damage to the skin, perpetuating the eczema cycle.

3. Systemic Inflammation: In severe cases, inflammation may not be limited to the skin. Some studies have found evidence of low-grade systemic inflammation in people with eczema, which may contribute to the increased risk of other health problems associated with the condition.

The inflammatory process in eczema involves a complex interplay of various cells and molecules:

- Cytokines: These signaling molecules coordinate the immune response. In eczema, there's often an overproduction of pro-inflammatory cytokines.

- Chemokines: These attract immune cells to the site of inflammation.

- Mast Cells: These release histamine and other inflammatory mediators.

- Eosinophils: These are often elevated in the blood and skin of people with eczema and contribute to inflammation.

Understanding this inflammatory cascade is crucial for developing targeted treatments, which we'll discuss in later chapters.

Conclusion: The Complex Web of Eczema

As we've explored in this chapter, eczema is a complex condition involving intricate interactions between the skin barrier, immune system, and genetic factors. From the compromised skin barrier to the overactive immune response, from genetic predisposition to environmental triggers, each aspect contributes to the development and persistence of eczema.

This complexity can seem overwhelming, but it also offers multiple points of intervention for treatment and management. By understanding the science behind eczema, we can better appreciate why certain treatments work and how lifestyle changes can make a significant difference.

Moreover, ongoing research into areas like genetics, the skin microbiome, and epigenetics is continually expanding our understanding of eczema. This research holds the promise of new, more targeted treatments in the future.

As we move forward in this book, we'll build on this scientific foundation to explore the various triggers of eczema, discuss diagnosis and assessment, and delve into both conventional and alternative treatment options. Armed with this knowledge, you'll be better equipped to manage eczema effectively and improve quality of life.

Remember, while the science of eczema is complex, you don't need to be a scientist to manage the condition effectively. In the coming chapters, we'll translate this scientific knowledge into practical strategies that you can apply in your daily life. Understanding the underlying mechanisms of eczema is just the first step on the journey to better skin health.

CHAPTER 3

Triggers and Risk Factors

Understanding the triggers and risk factors associated with eczema is crucial for effective management of the condition. In this chapter, we'll explore the various elements that can provoke or exacerbate eczema symptoms, as well as the factors that may increase an individual's likelihood of developing the condition. By identifying these triggers and risk factors, we can develop more targeted strategies for prevention and treatment.

Environmental Triggers

Environmental factors play a significant role in triggering or worsening eczema symptoms. These can vary from person to person, but some common environmental triggers include:

1. Weather Conditions:
   - Cold, dry weather can lead to skin dryness and irritation.
   - Hot, humid conditions can cause sweating, which may irritate the skin.
   - Sudden temperature changes can also trigger flare-ups.

2. Air Quality:
   - Air pollution, including particulate matter and volatile organic compounds, can irritate the skin.
   - Tobacco smoke, both firsthand and secondhand, can exacerbate eczema

symptoms.

3. Water Hardness:
   - Hard water, which contains high levels of minerals like calcium and magnesium, can dry out the skin and potentially worsen eczema.
   - Some studies suggest that living in areas with hard water may increase the risk of developing eczema in early life.

4. UV Radiation:
   - While sunlight can sometimes improve eczema symptoms, excessive sun exposure can lead to skin damage and trigger flare-ups in some individuals.

5. Indoor Environment:
   - Dust mites, a common allergen found in homes, can trigger eczema symptoms in sensitive individuals.
   - Mold spores, which thrive in damp environments, can also be a trigger.

6. Occupational Exposures:
   - Certain professions that involve frequent hand-washing or exposure to irritants (e.g., healthcare workers, hairdressers, mechanics) may be at higher risk for hand eczema.

Managing environmental triggers often involves a combination of avoidance strategies and protective measures. This might include using a humidifier in dry environments, protecting the skin from extreme weather conditions, and maintaining good indoor air quality.

Allergens and Irritants

Allergens and irritants are substances that can trigger an immune response or directly irritate the skin, leading to eczema flare-ups. These can be broadly categorized into two groups:

Allergens:
   1. Food Allergens:
   - Common food allergens include milk, eggs, peanuts, tree nuts, soy, wheat, and fish.
   - While food allergies don't cause eczema, they can trigger flare-ups in some people, particularly children.

2. Airborne Allergens:
   - Pollen from trees, grasses, and weeds
   - Animal dander
   - Dust mites
   - Mold spores

3. Contact Allergens:
   - Metals, particularly nickel
   - Fragrances in personal care products and cleaning supplies
   - Certain fabrics, like wool or synthetic fibers
   - Latex

Irritants:
   1. Soaps and Detergents:
   - Harsh soaps, particularly those with high pH levels, can strip the skin of its natural oils.
   - Laundry detergents, especially those with fragrances or dyes, can irritate sensitive skin.

2. Clothing:
   - Rough or scratchy fabrics like wool can irritate the skin.
   - Tight clothing that doesn't allow the skin to breathe can lead to overheating and sweating.

3. Personal Care Products:
   - Products containing alcohol, fragrances, or other potential irritants can

trigger flare-ups.
   - Even some products marketed for sensitive skin may contain ingredients that irritate some individuals.

4. Household Cleaning Products:
   - Many cleaning products contain harsh chemicals that can irritate the skin.

5. Metals:
   - Nickel, found in jewelry, belt buckles, and even some foods, is a common trigger for contact dermatitis.

6. Plants:
   - Some plants, like poison ivy or stinging nettles, can cause skin reactions in many people.

Identifying specific allergens and irritants can be challenging, as reactions may be delayed and can vary from person to person. Keeping a detailed diary of exposures and symptoms can help identify patterns. In some cases, allergy testing may be recommended to pinpoint specific triggers.

Stress and Emotional Factors

The link between stress and eczema is well-established, though the exact mechanisms are still being studied. Stress can trigger or exacerbate eczema symptoms in several ways:

1. Immune System Effects:
   - Stress can alter immune function, potentially increasing inflammation in the body.
   - This can lead to increased production of stress hormones like cortisol, which can affect skin health.

2. Skin Barrier Function:
  - Stress may impair the skin's barrier function, making it more susceptible to irritants and allergens.

3. Behavioral Changes:
  - Stress can lead to changes in behavior, such as decreased attention to skincare routines or increased scratching.

4. Sleep Disruption:
  - Stress often interferes with sleep, which can in turn affect skin health and healing.

5. Neurogenic Inflammation:
  - Stress can trigger the release of neuropeptides in the skin, leading to inflammation and itching.

Other emotional factors can also play a role in eczema:

- Anxiety: Can lead to increased itching and scratching behaviors.
  - Depression: May result in neglect of skincare routines and overall health.
  - Frustration: The chronic nature of eczema can lead to frustration, potentially exacerbating symptoms.

Managing stress and emotional wellbeing is an important aspect of eczema care. Techniques such as mindfulness, cognitive-behavioral therapy, and stress-reduction practices can be beneficial for many individuals with eczema.

Hormonal Factors

Hormones can play a significant role in eczema, particularly for women. Hormonal changes can affect skin hydration, oil production, and immune function, potentially triggering or exacerbating eczema symptoms.

Key hormonal factors include:

1. Menstrual Cycle:
   - Some women experience eczema flare-ups at specific points in their menstrual cycle, often correlating with changes in estrogen and progesterone levels.

2. Pregnancy:
   - Pregnancy can have variable effects on eczema. Some women experience improvement, while others may see worsening of symptoms.
   - Postpartum hormonal changes can also trigger flare-ups.

3. Menopause:
   - The hormonal changes associated with menopause can lead to increased skin dryness and sensitivity, potentially exacerbating eczema.

4. Thyroid Hormones:
   - Both hypothyroidism and hyperthyroidism can affect skin health and potentially influence eczema symptoms.

5. Stress Hormones:
   - As mentioned earlier, stress hormones like cortisol can affect skin health and immune function.

Understanding these hormonal influences can help in predicting and managing flare-ups. In some cases, hormonal therapies may be considered as part of a comprehensive eczema management plan.

Dietary Factors

The relationship between diet and eczema is complex and often individualized. While food allergies can certainly trigger eczema symptoms in some individuals, the role of diet in eczema goes beyond just allergies.

Potential dietary influences on eczema include:

1. Food Allergies:
   - As mentioned earlier, common food allergens like milk, eggs, and nuts can trigger eczema flare-ups in allergic individuals.

2. Food Sensitivities:
   - Some people may have non-allergic food sensitivities that can exacerbate eczema symptoms.
   - Common culprits include dairy, gluten, and certain preservatives or additives.

3. Nutritional Deficiencies:
   - Deficiencies in certain nutrients may contribute to skin health issues. Key nutrients include:
   - Omega-3 fatty acids: Important for skin barrier function and reducing inflammation.
   - Vitamin D: Plays a role in skin health and immune function.
   - Zinc: Important for wound healing and immune function.
   - Vitamin E: An antioxidant that supports skin health.

4. Histamine-Rich Foods:
   - Some people with eczema may be sensitive to histamine-rich foods, which can potentially trigger symptoms.
   - These include fermented foods, aged cheeses, and certain fruits and vegetables.

5. Inflammatory Foods:
   - Foods that promote inflammation in the body may potentially exacerbate eczema symptoms.
   - These often include processed foods, foods high in sugar, and certain types of fats.

6. Probiotics and Gut Health:
   - There's growing evidence suggesting a link between gut health and skin health.
   - Some studies have shown potential benefits of probiotic supplementation in managing eczema, particularly in children.

It's important to note that dietary triggers can be highly individual. What triggers symptoms in one person may not affect another. Keeping a food diary and working with a healthcare provider or registered dietitian can help identify potential dietary triggers or deficiencies.

Genetic Risk Factors

While we touched on genetics in the previous chapter, it's worth exploring genetic risk factors in more detail here. Genetic predisposition is a significant risk factor for developing eczema, particularly atopic dermatitis.

Key genetic factors include:

1. Family History:
   - Having a parent or sibling with eczema significantly increases an individual's risk of developing the condition.
   - The risk is even higher if both parents have eczema or other atopic conditions.

2. Specific Gene Mutations:
   - Filaggrin (FLG) Gene: Mutations in this gene, which is crucial for skin barrier function, are strongly associated with atopic dermatitis.
   - Immune System Genes: Variations in genes related to immune function, such as those involved in T cell function or cytokine production, can increase eczema risk.
   - Skin Barrier Genes: Beyond filaggrin, mutations in other genes involved in skin barrier function (like SPINK5) can increase susceptibility to eczema.

3. Atopic Tendency:
 - Individuals with a genetic predisposition to atopic conditions (eczema, asthma, allergic rhinitis) are at higher risk.

4. Ethnic Background:
 - Some studies suggest that eczema prevalence may vary among different ethnic groups, which may be partly due to genetic factors.

Understanding genetic risk factors can be helpful for early intervention and prevention strategies, particularly in high-risk infants. However, it's important to remember that having genetic risk factors doesn't guarantee that an individual will develop eczema. Environmental factors and gene-environment interactions also play crucial roles.

Microbiome Imbalance

The role of the microbiome in eczema is an area of active research. The skin microbiome, which we introduced in the previous chapter, can be a significant factor in eczema development and severity.

Key points about microbiome imbalance in eczema include:

1. Reduced Diversity:
 - People with eczema often have less diverse skin microbiomes compared to those without the condition.
 - This reduced diversity may make the skin more susceptible to colonization by harmful bacteria.

2. Staphylococcus aureus Overgrowth:
 - S. aureus is often found in higher numbers on eczematous skin.
 - This bacteria can produce toxins that trigger inflammation and damage the skin barrier.

3. Beneficial Bacteria Deficiency:
   - Certain bacteria, like some strains of Staphylococcus epidermidis, may help protect against eczema.
   - These beneficial bacteria are often found in lower numbers in people with eczema.

4. Gut Microbiome Connection:
   - There's growing evidence suggesting a link between gut microbiome health and skin conditions, including eczema.
   - Imbalances in the gut microbiome (dysbiosis) may contribute to systemic inflammation and immune dysfunction.

Factors that can influence microbiome balance include:
   - Antibiotic use, especially in early life
   - Diet
   - Environmental exposures
   - Use of certain skincare products

Understanding the role of the microbiome opens up new avenues for eczema prevention and treatment, including the potential use of probiotics (both topical and oral) and strategies to promote a healthy, diverse microbiome.

Age and Developmental Stages

Eczema can affect individuals at any age, but it often follows certain patterns related to age and developmental stages:

1. Infancy (0-2 years):
   - Eczema often first appears in infancy, typically around 3-6 months of age.
   - It commonly affects the face, scalp, and extensor surfaces of the arms and legs.
   - Food allergies may play a more significant role in triggering eczema at

this age.

2. Childhood (2-12 years):
   - Eczema may persist from infancy or develop during childhood.
   - It often affects the flexural areas (inside of elbows, behind knees).
   - Environmental allergens become more significant triggers.

3. Adolescence and Adulthood:
   - Some individuals may experience improvement or resolution of eczema during adolescence.
   - For others, eczema may persist into adulthood or even develop for the first time (adult-onset eczema).
   - Occupational exposures and stress often become more significant factors.

4. Elderly:
   - Eczema in the elderly may be complicated by age-related changes in the skin, including decreased barrier function and slower healing.
   - Certain types of eczema, like asteatotic eczema, are more common in older adults.

Understanding these age-related patterns can help in predicting the course of eczema and tailoring management strategies appropriately.

Geographic and Socioeconomic Factors

Geographic location and socioeconomic status can influence eczema risk and severity in several ways:

1. Climate:
   - Eczema prevalence tends to be higher in countries with cooler climates.
   - However, rapidly changing climate conditions may be altering these patterns.

2. Urban vs. Rural Environment:
   - Eczema rates are generally higher in urban areas compared to rural areas.
   - This may be due to differences in pollution levels, lifestyle factors, or exposure to certain allergens.

3. Socioeconomic Status:
   - The relationship between socioeconomic status and eczema is complex and can vary by region.
   - In some areas, higher socioeconomic status is associated with increased eczema risk (the "hygiene hypothesis").
   - In other regions, lower socioeconomic status may be associated with increased risk, possibly due to factors like overcrowding or reduced access to healthcare.

4. Access to Healthcare:
   - Disparities in access to healthcare can affect eczema diagnosis, treatment, and overall management.

5. Cultural Practices:
   - Cultural differences in diet, lifestyle, and skincare practices can influence eczema risk and management.

Understanding these geographic and socioeconomic factors is important for developing public health strategies and for healthcare providers in tailoring their approach to diverse patient populations.

Conclusion: The Multifaceted Nature of Eczema Triggers and Risk Factors

As we've explored in this chapter, the triggers and risk factors for eczema are diverse and often interconnected. From environmental allergens to genetic predisposition, from hormonal fluctuations to microbiome imbalances, each factor plays a role in the complex tapestry of eczema development and exacerbation.

Understanding these triggers and risk factors is crucial for several reasons:

1. Personalized Management: By identifying individual triggers, people with eczema can develop personalized strategies to avoid or mitigate flare-ups.

2. Prevention: Understanding risk factors can help in developing prevention strategies, particularly for high-risk individuals.

3. Treatment Approaches: Knowledge of triggers and risk factors informs treatment approaches, allowing for more targeted interventions.

4. Research Directions: This understanding guides researchers in developing new treatments and prevention strategies.

5. Patient Empowerment: When individuals understand their eczema triggers and risk factors, they're better equipped to take an active role in managing their condition.

It's important to remember that eczema triggers and risk factors can be highly individual. What provokes symptoms in one person may not affect another. Therefore, a personalized approach to identifying and managing triggers is crucial.

In the next chapters, we'll build on this understanding as we explore diagnosis, treatment options, and management strategies. By combining knowledge of triggers and risk factors with effective treatment approaches, individuals with eczema can work towards better control of their symptoms and improved quality of life.

CHAPTER 4

Diagnosis and Medical Assessment

Accurate diagnosis and comprehensive medical assessment are crucial first steps in effectively managing eczema. In this chapter, we'll explore the process of diagnosing eczema, including the criteria used by healthcare professionals, the various tests that may be employed, and the importance of differential diagnosis. We'll also discuss how the severity of eczema is assessed and the role of ongoing monitoring in managing this chronic condition.

The Diagnostic Process

Diagnosing eczema, particularly atopic dermatitis, is primarily a clinical process. This means that healthcare providers rely heavily on the patient's medical history and physical examination rather than specific laboratory tests. However, additional tests may be used to rule out other conditions or identify potential triggers.

1. Medical History

The first step in diagnosing eczema is a thorough medical history. The healthcare provider will typically ask about:

- Symptoms: The nature, duration, and frequency of symptoms such as itching, redness, and dry skin.

- Family history: Whether there's a history of eczema, asthma, or allergies in close family members.

- Potential triggers: Any noticed patterns related to flare-ups, such as exposure to certain substances or stressful events.

- Impact on daily life: How symptoms affect sleep, work or school performance, and overall quality of life.

- Previous treatments: What treatments have been tried and their effectiveness.

- Other medical conditions: Particularly other skin conditions or allergic disorders.

2. Physical Examination

A thorough physical examination is crucial for diagnosing eczema. The healthcare provider will look for characteristic signs of eczema, including:

- Dry, scaly skin
  - Redness (erythema)
  - Swelling (edema)
  - Crusting or oozing
  - Lichenification (thickened skin due to chronic scratching)
  - Specific distribution patterns typical of eczema (e.g., flexural areas in atopic dermatitis)

The provider will also assess the extent of affected areas and the overall severity of the condition.

Diagnostic Criteria

While there's no single definitive test for eczema, several sets of diagnostic criteria have been developed to aid in diagnosis. One widely used set is the Hanifin and Rajka criteria for atopic dermatitis, which includes:

Major Features (must have three or more):
- Pruritus (itching)
- Typical morphology and distribution (e.g., flexural lichenification in adults)
- Chronic or chronically relapsing dermatitis
- Personal or family history of atopy (eczema, asthma, allergic rhinitis)

Minor Features (must have three or more):
- Xerosis (dry skin)
- Ichthyosis (scaly skin) / palmar hyperlinearity / keratosis pilaris
- Immediate (type I) skin test reactivity
- Elevated serum IgE
- Early age of onset
- Tendency toward cutaneous infections
- Tendency toward non-specific hand or foot dermatitis
- Nipple eczema
- Cheilitis (lip inflammation)
- Recurrent conjunctivitis
- Dennie-Morgan infraorbital fold
- Keratoconus (conical cornea)
- Anterior subcapsular cataracts
- Orbital darkening
- Facial pallor / facial erythema
- Pityriasis alba (white patches on the face)
- Anterior neck folds
- Itch when sweating
- Intolerance to wool and lipid solvents
- Perifollicular accentuation
- Food intolerance
- Course influenced by environmental / emotional factors
- White dermographism / delayed blanch

It's important to note that not all of these features need to be present for a diagnosis of atopic dermatitis. The diagnosis is based on the overall clinical picture.

Additional Diagnostic Tests

While not always necessary, certain tests may be used to support the diagnosis or rule out other conditions:

1. Allergy Tests:
   - Skin prick tests or blood tests (specific IgE) may be used to identify potential allergen triggers.
   - Patch tests can help identify contact allergens in cases of suspected allergic contact dermatitis.

2. Skin Biopsy:
   - While rarely necessary for typical cases of eczema, a skin biopsy may be performed if the diagnosis is uncertain or to rule out other conditions.

3. Blood Tests:
   - Complete blood count (CBC) may be done to check for elevated eosinophils, which are often seen in atopic conditions.
   - Serum IgE levels may be measured, as they are often elevated in atopic dermatitis.

4. Skin Barrier Function Tests:
   - Transepidermal water loss (TEWL) measurement can assess skin barrier function.
   - pH measurement of the skin surface can provide information about skin barrier health.

5. Microbial Cultures:
   - If secondary infection is suspected, cultures may be taken to identify the causative organism.

Differential Diagnosis

Eczema can sometimes be confused with other skin conditions. Part of the diagnostic process involves ruling out these other conditions, known as differential diagnosis. Some conditions that may need to be considered include:

1. Psoriasis: Can sometimes resemble eczema, particularly in certain locations like the scalp.

2. Seborrheic Dermatitis: Often affects similar areas to eczema, particularly in infants (cradle cap).

3. Contact Dermatitis: Can be difficult to distinguish from atopic dermatitis, especially if the contact allergen is not obvious.

4. Scabies: Can cause intense itching and rash that may resemble eczema.

5. Fungal Infections: Certain fungal skin infections can mimic eczema.

6. Cutaneous T-cell Lymphoma: In rare cases, this type of skin lymphoma can resemble chronic eczema.

7. Nutritional Deficiencies: Certain vitamin deficiencies can cause skin changes that may be mistaken for eczema.

8. Other Less Common Conditions: Various other skin conditions, such as ichthyosis or immunodeficiency disorders, may need to be considered in atypical cases.

Accurate differentiation between these conditions is crucial for appropriate treatment. In some cases, a person may have more than one condition simultaneously, further complicating the diagnosis.

Assessing Eczema Severity

Once eczema is diagnosed, assessing its severity is important for determining the appropriate treatment approach and monitoring progress over time. Several scoring systems have been developed for this purpose:

1. SCORAD (SCORing Atopic Dermatitis):
   This widely used system assesses three components:
   - Extent: The percentage of body surface area affected
   - Intensity: The severity of six clinical signs (redness, swelling, ooz-ing/crusting, excoriation, skin thickening, and dryness)
   - Subjective symptoms: The impact on sleep and itching

2. EASI (Eczema Area and Severity Index):
   This system focuses on objective measures, assessing four clinical signs (redness, thickness, scratching, and lichenification) in four body regions.

3. Patient-Oriented Eczema Measure (POEM):
   This tool focuses on the patient's experience, asking about the frequency of seven symptoms over the past week.

4. Investigator's Global Assessment (IGA):
   A simple scale where the healthcare provider rates the overall severity of eczema from clear to severe.

These scoring systems help in:
   - Standardizing assessment across different healthcare providers
   - Monitoring changes in severity over time
   - Evaluating the effectiveness of treatments
   - Determining eligibility for certain treatments, particularly in research settings

It's worth noting that eczema severity can fluctuate over time, and regular reassessment is often necessary.

Specialized Assessments

In some cases, particularly for more severe or treatment-resistant eczema, additional specialized assessments may be warranted:

1. Patch Testing:
   For suspected allergic contact dermatitis, patch testing involves applying potential allergens to the skin under patches and observing for reactions over several days.

2. Photo Testing:
   If photosensitivity is suspected, controlled exposure to different wavelengths of light can help identify light-sensitive eczema.

3. Nutritional Assessment:
   In cases where dietary factors are suspected to play a significant role, a detailed nutritional assessment may be helpful.

4. Psychological Assessment:
   Given the significant impact eczema can have on mental health, psychological evaluation may be appropriate in some cases.

5. Occupational Assessment:
   For individuals with suspected occupational eczema, a detailed review of workplace exposures may be necessary.

The Role of Specialist Referral

While many cases of eczema can be managed by primary care providers, referral to a specialist may be necessary in certain situations:

1. Dermatologist:
   - For difficult-to-control eczema
   - When the diagnosis is uncertain
   - For consideration of advanced therapies

2. Allergist/Immunologist:
   - For comprehensive allergy testing
   - When multiple allergic conditions are present (e.g., eczema with asthma and food allergies)

3. Pediatric Specialist:
   - For young children with severe or treatment-resistant eczema

4. Occupational Health Specialist:
   - For suspected work-related eczema

5. Mental Health Professional:
   - When eczema is significantly impacting mental health and quality of life

Ongoing Monitoring and Follow-up

Eczema is a chronic condition that requires ongoing monitoring and management. Regular follow-up is important for several reasons:

1. Assessing Treatment Effectiveness:
   Regular check-ups allow healthcare providers to evaluate how well current treatments are working and make adjustments as needed.

2. Monitoring for Side Effects:
   Some eczema treatments, particularly long-term use of topical corticosteroids or systemic medications, require monitoring for potential side effects.

3. Catching Complications Early:

Regular examinations can help identify and address complications like skin infections promptly.

4. Adjusting Management Strategies:
As eczema can change over time, regular follow-up allows for timely adjustments to management strategies.

5. Providing Ongoing Education and Support:
Follow-up visits provide opportunities for ongoing patient education and support, which are crucial for successful long-term management.

The frequency of follow-up will depend on the severity of eczema and the types of treatments being used. It may range from several times a year for severe cases to annual check-ups for well-controlled eczema.

The Importance of Self-Monitoring

While regular medical follow-up is important, self-monitoring plays a crucial role in day-to-day eczema management. Patients (or parents of children with eczema) should be encouraged to:

1. Keep a Symptom Diary:
Tracking symptoms, potential triggers, and treatment use can provide valuable insights and help inform treatment decisions.

2. Regularly Assess Skin Condition:
Developing the habit of regularly examining the skin can help catch flare-ups early.

3. Monitor Treatment Use:
Keeping track of medication use, particularly topical corticosteroids, is important for safe and effective management.

4. Track Quality of Life Impact:

Noting how eczema affects daily activities, sleep, and emotional well-being can help in assessing the overall impact of the condition.

Emerging Diagnostic Tools

As our understanding of eczema grows and technology advances, new diagnostic tools are emerging:

1. Genetic Testing:

While not routinely used in clinical practice, genetic testing for mutations associated with eczema (like filaggrin gene mutations) may become more common in the future, particularly for research purposes.

2. Tape Stripping:

This minimally invasive technique involves applying and removing adhesive tape from the skin surface to collect samples for analysis of biomarkers.

3. Skin Microbiome Analysis:

As we learn more about the role of the skin microbiome in eczema, techniques for analyzing the microbial composition of the skin may become more widely used.

4. Advanced Imaging Techniques:

Technologies like confocal microscopy may offer new ways to assess skin structure and function non-invasively.

5. Artificial Intelligence:

Machine learning algorithms are being developed to assist in eczema diagnosis and severity assessment based on digital images of the skin.

While these emerging tools show promise, it's important to note that clinical assessment by a healthcare professional remains the gold standard for eczema diagnosis and management.

Conclusion: The Cornerstone of Effective Eczema Management

Accurate diagnosis and comprehensive assessment form the foundation of effective eczema management. By combining careful clinical evaluation with appropriate diagnostic tests and severity assessments, healthcare providers can develop tailored treatment plans that address each individual's unique needs.

For individuals with eczema and their caregivers, understanding the diagnostic process can help in several ways:

1. It empowers patients to provide relevant information to their healthcare providers, facilitating more accurate diagnosis.

2. It helps set realistic expectations about the diagnostic process and the ongoing nature of eczema management.

3. It underscores the importance of regular follow-up and self-monitoring in managing this chronic condition.

4. It provides a framework for understanding how treatment decisions are made and how progress is evaluated.

As we move forward in this book to discuss treatment options and management strategies, keep in mind that these approaches are built upon the foundation of accurate diagnosis and ongoing assessment. By partnering with healthcare providers and actively participating in the diagnostic and monitoring process, individuals with eczema can play a crucial role in optimizing their care and improving their quality of life.

CHAPTER 5

onventional Treatments

Having explored the diagnosis and assessment of eczema in the previous chapter, we now turn our attention to the various conventional treatments available. These evidence-based approaches form the backbone of eczema management in modern medicine. In this chapter, we'll discuss topical treatments, systemic medications, and phototherapy, examining their benefits, potential side effects, and appropriate use.

Topical Treatments

Topical treatments are the first line of defense against eczema and are often sufficient to manage mild to moderate cases. They are applied directly to the skin and come in various forms, including creams, ointments, lotions, and gels.

1. Emollients and Moisturizers

Emollients and moisturizers are the foundation of eczema treatment and should be used regularly, even when the skin is not actively inflamed.

Benefits:
- Improve skin hydration
- Strengthen the skin barrier

- Reduce itching and inflammation
- Help prevent flare-ups

Types:
- Ointments: Most occlusive, best for very dry skin
- Creams: Less greasy, good for everyday use
- Lotions: Lightest, suitable for hairy areas but less moisturizing

Key ingredients may include:
- Ceramides: Help restore the skin barrier
- Hyaluronic acid: Attracts and retains moisture
- Glycerin: Helps skin retain moisture
- Petrolatum: Creates a protective barrier

Usage:
- Apply liberally at least twice daily
- Best applied after bathing, while skin is still damp

2. Topical Corticosteroids

Topical corticosteroids are anti-inflammatory medications and are the mainstay of treatment for eczema flare-ups.

Benefits:
- Reduce inflammation
- Relieve itching
- Help heal the skin

Types:
- Range from mild (e.g., hydrocortisone) to very potent (e.g., clobetasol)
- Come in various formulations: creams, ointments, lotions, foams

Usage:

- Applied to inflamed areas during flare-ups
- Frequency and duration depend on strength and location
- Often used in a "step-down" approach, starting with a stronger steroid and gradually moving to milder ones

Potential side effects:
- Skin thinning (atrophy)
- Stretch marks
- Changes in skin pigmentation
- Rarely, systemic effects if overused

To minimize side effects:
- Use the lowest effective strength
- Follow prescribed regimen
- Use intermittently rather than continuously
- Be cautious in sensitive areas (face, genitals)

3. Topical Calcineurin Inhibitors (TCIs)

TCIs, such as tacrolimus and pimecrolimus, are non-steroidal anti-inflammatory medications.

Benefits:
- Reduce inflammation and itching
- Can be used long-term
- Don't cause skin thinning
- Suitable for sensitive areas like the face and eyelids

Usage:
- Applied twice daily during flare-ups
- Can be used for maintenance therapy to prevent flares

Potential side effects:

- Burning or stinging sensation upon application (usually temporary)
- Increased risk of skin infections

Note: TCIs carry a "black box" warning about a theoretical risk of skin cancer and lymphoma, but long-term studies have not shown an increased risk.

4. Topical PDE4 Inhibitors

Crisaborole is a phosphodiesterase 4 (PDE4) inhibitor approved for mild to moderate atopic dermatitis.

Benefits:
- Reduces inflammation
- Can be used long-term
- Suitable for sensitive areas

Usage:
- Applied twice daily to affected areas

Potential side effects:
- Burning or stinging at the application site

5. Topical Antibiotics

Used when there's evidence of secondary bacterial infection.

Common options:
- Mupirocin
- Fusidic acid

Usage:
- Applied to affected areas, usually for a short duration

Note: Overuse can lead to antibiotic resistance, so these should be used judiciously.

6. Wet Wrap Therapy

This technique involves applying topical medications and moisturizers, then wrapping the area with wet bandages followed by dry ones.

Benefits:
  - Increases effectiveness of topical treatments
  - Provides intense hydration
  - Helps calm severe flares

Usage:
  - Typically done under healthcare provider guidance
  - Can be used for short periods during severe flares

Systemic Medications

For severe or widespread eczema that doesn't respond adequately to topical treatments, systemic medications may be necessary. These are taken orally or by injection and work throughout the body.

1. Oral Corticosteroids

Oral corticosteroids, such as prednisone, are powerful anti-inflammatory medications.

Benefits:
  - Quickly reduce inflammation and itching in severe flares

Usage:
  - Usually prescribed for short courses (1-3 weeks)

- Typically used as a "rescue" treatment for severe flares

Potential side effects:
  - Weight gain
  - Mood changes
  - Increased risk of infections
  - Long-term use can lead to osteoporosis, diabetes, and other serious side effects

Note: Due to potential side effects, oral corticosteroids are not recommended for long-term use in eczema management.

2. Immunosuppressants

For severe, chronic eczema, immunosuppressant medications may be prescribed.

Common options:
  - Cyclosporine
  - Methotrexate
  - Azathioprine
  - Mycophenolate mofetil

Benefits:
  - Can provide significant improvement in severe cases
  - May allow reduction in topical corticosteroid use

Potential side effects:
  - Increased risk of infections
  - Nausea and other gastrointestinal symptoms
  - Liver and kidney effects (require monitoring)
  - Long-term use may increase risk of certain cancers

Usage:
  - Typically used for limited periods under close medical supervision
  - Regular blood tests are required to monitor for side effects

3. Biologic Drugs

Biologic drugs are a newer class of medications that target specific parts of the immune system involved in eczema.

Dupilumab:
  - The first biologic approved for moderate to severe atopic dermatitis
  - Targets interleukin-4 and interleukin-13, key drivers of inflammation in eczema

Benefits:
  - Can provide significant improvement in severe cases
  - May improve associated symptoms like asthma and nasal polyps

Usage:
  - Given by subcutaneous injection every two weeks

Potential side effects:
  - Injection site reactions
  - Eye inflammation (conjunctivitis)
  - Rarely, severe allergic reactions

Other biologics:
  - Several other biologics targeting different aspects of the immune response in eczema are in development or newly approved

4. JAK Inhibitors

Janus kinase (JAK) inhibitors are a newer class of oral medications for moderate to severe atopic dermatitis.

Options:
- Upadacitinib
- Abrocitinib
- Baricitinib

Benefits:
- Can provide rapid and significant improvement
- Oral administration (unlike biologics)

Potential side effects:
- Increased risk of infections
- Changes in blood cell counts
- Rare but serious side effects including blood clots and certain cancers

Usage:
- Taken orally, usually once daily
- Require regular monitoring due to potential side effects

5. Antihistamines

While not directly treating the inflammation in eczema, antihistamines can help manage itching.

Benefits:
- Reduce itching, especially at night
- May improve sleep

Types:
- Sedating (e.g., diphenhydramine): Can be helpful for nighttime itching
- Non-sedating (e.g., cetirizine, fexofenadine): Less likely to cause drowsiness

Usage:
- Can be used as needed or regularly
- Choice depends on individual response and timing of symptoms

6. Antibiotics

Oral antibiotics may be prescribed if there's evidence of widespread secondary bacterial infection.

Common options:
- Flucloxacillin
- Erythromycin
- Cephalexin

Usage:
- Usually prescribed for short courses (1-2 weeks)
- Choice depends on likely causative bacteria and local resistance patterns

Phototherapy

Phototherapy, or light therapy, involves exposing the skin to specific wavelengths of ultraviolet (UV) light under medical supervision.

Types:

1. Narrowband UVB: Most commonly used, effective and relatively safe
2. Broadband UVB: Less commonly used now
3. UVA1: May be used for severe cases
4. PUVA (Psoralen + UVA): Less commonly used due to higher risks

Benefits:
- Reduces inflammation

- Can provide long-lasting improvement
- May reduce bacterial load on the skin

Potential side effects:
   - Short-term: Redness, burning
   - Long-term: Premature skin aging, increased skin cancer risk (especially with PUVA)

Usage:
   - Typically 2-3 sessions per week for several weeks
   - Gradually increasing exposure times
   - Often used in combination with topical treatments
   - May be used for maintenance therapy

Considerations:
   - Requires commitment to regular treatments
   - May not be suitable for all skin types
   - Long-term risks need to be weighed against benefits

Combination Approaches

In practice, eczema management often involves a combination of treatments. This may include:

- Daily use of emollients
   - Topical anti-inflammatory treatments for flares
   - Occasional use of systemic medications for severe flares
   - Antihistamines for itch control
   - Phototherapy for widespread disease or maintenance

The specific combination will depend on the individual's eczema severity, distribution, and response to treatments.

Treatment Challenges and Considerations

While these conventional treatments can be very effective, there are several challenges to consider:

1. Adherence: Many treatments, particularly topical ones, require consistent, sometimes multiple daily applications. This can be challenging for many patients.

2. Corticosteroid Phobia: Fear of side effects from topical corticosteroids can lead to underuse and poor control.

3. Cost: Some newer treatments, particularly biologics, can be very expensive and may not be covered by all insurance plans.

4. Long-term Safety: The long-term safety of newer treatments is still being studied.

5. Individual Variation: Response to treatments can vary significantly between individuals.

6. Impact on Quality of Life: Some treatments may be burdensome or have side effects that impact quality of life.

7. Pediatric Considerations: Treatment choices may be more limited in young children, and long-term safety is particularly important.

8. Pregnancy and Breastfeeding: Many treatments have limited safety data in pregnancy and breastfeeding.

Emerging Treatments

The field of eczema treatment is rapidly evolving, with several new approaches in development:

1. New Biologics: Several new biologics targeting different aspects of the immune response are in clinical trials.

2. Topical JAK Inhibitors: These may provide a new option for topical anti-inflammatory treatment.

3. Microbiome-based Therapies: Treatments aimed at modulating the skin microbiome are being investigated.

4. Barrier Repair Therapies: New approaches to improve skin barrier function are in development.

5. Targeted Therapies: As we understand more about the different subtypes of eczema, more targeted therapies may become available.

The Role of the Healthcare Provider

Given the complexity of eczema management and the range of available treatments, the role of the healthcare provider is crucial. They can:

- Develop an individualized treatment plan
  - Adjust treatments based on response
  - Monitor for side effects
  - Provide education on proper use of treatments
  - Address concerns and misconceptions
  - Stay updated on new treatment options

The Importance of Patient Education

For successful eczema management, patient education is key. This includes:

- Understanding how to use treatments correctly
    - Recognizing when to seek medical attention
    - Understanding the chronic nature of eczema and the need for ongoing management
    - Being aware of potential side effects and how to minimize them
    - Learning about lifestyle measures that can complement medical treatments

Conclusion: A Toolkit for Eczema Management

Conventional treatments for eczema offer a diverse toolkit for managing this challenging condition. From daily moisturizing to powerful systemic medications, these treatments can help control symptoms, prevent flares, and improve quality of life for many people with eczema.

However, it's important to remember that eczema management is often a process of trial and error. What works best can vary from person to person and may change over time. Patience, persistence, and good communication with healthcare providers are key to finding the most effective treatment approach.

Moreover, while these treatments can be very effective, they are most successful when combined with good skincare practices, trigger avoidance, and lifestyle measures. In the next chapter, we'll explore these complementary approaches to eczema management, providing a holistic view of how to live well with this chronic condition.

As research continues and new treatments emerge, the future looks bright for eczema management. However, the foundation remains the same: a personalized approach, consistent care, and a strong partnership between patients and their healthcare providers.

CHAPTER 6

Natural and Alternative Therapies

While conventional treatments form the backbone of eczema management, many individuals seek natural and alternative therapies to complement their treatment regimen or as alternatives to traditional medications. In this chapter, we'll explore various natural remedies, complementary therapies, and alternative approaches to managing eczema. It's important to note that while some of these methods show promise, the scientific evidence supporting their efficacy varies. Always consult with a healthcare provider before incorporating new treatments into your eczema management plan.

Herbal Remedies

Herbal remedies have been used for centuries to treat various skin conditions, including eczema. While scientific evidence is limited for many of these treatments, some show promise in managing eczema symptoms.

1. Chamomile:
   - Anti-inflammatory and soothing properties
   - Can be used as a topical application or tea
   - Some studies suggest it may be as effective as low-potency hydrocortisone for mild eczema

2. Aloe Vera:
  - Known for its soothing and moisturizing effects
  - May help reduce inflammation and itching
  - Can be applied topically as a gel or cream

3. Calendula:
  - Has anti-inflammatory and wound-healing properties
  - Often used in creams or ointments for eczema
  - May help soothe irritated skin and promote healing

4. Evening Primrose Oil:
  - Contains gamma-linolenic acid (GLA), an omega-6 fatty acid
  - Some studies suggest oral supplementation may help improve eczema symptoms
  - Results are mixed, and more research is needed

5. Borage Oil:
  - Another source of GLA
  - Some studies show promise for reducing eczema symptoms, but results are inconsistent

6. Witch Hazel:
  - Has astringent and anti-inflammatory properties
  - May help soothe itching and reduce inflammation
  - Can be applied topically as a compress or in creams

7. Licorice Root:
  - Contains compounds with anti-inflammatory effects
  - May help reduce itching and inflammation
  - Often used in topical preparations for eczema

8. St. John's Wort:
  - Has anti-inflammatory properties

- Some studies suggest topical application may help reduce eczema symptoms
    - Caution: Can increase sun sensitivity

It's important to note that herbal remedies can cause allergic reactions or interact with other medications. Always patch test before using a new product and consult with a healthcare provider, especially if you're pregnant, breastfeeding, or taking other medications.

Essential Oils

Essential oils are concentrated plant extracts that are sometimes used in eczema management. While some people find them helpful, it's crucial to use them properly as they can cause skin irritation if used incorrectly.

1. Tea Tree Oil:
    - Has antimicrobial properties
    - May help reduce inflammation and itching
    - Should always be diluted before application

2. Lavender Oil:
    - Known for its calming and anti-inflammatory properties
    - May help reduce stress, which can trigger eczema flares
    - Can be used in aromatherapy or diluted for topical use

3. German Chamomile Oil:
    - Contains chamazulene, which has anti-inflammatory properties
    - May help soothe irritated skin
    - Should be diluted before use

4. Geranium Oil:
    - Has anti-inflammatory and antimicrobial properties
    - May help balance sebum production

- Should be diluted before application

5. Frankincense Oil:
   - Known for its anti-inflammatory properties
   - May help reduce scarring and promote skin healing
   - Should be diluted before use

When using essential oils:
   - Always dilute in a carrier oil (like coconut oil or jojoba oil) before applying to the skin
   - Perform a patch test before widespread use
   - Avoid using on broken or severely inflamed skin
   - Be aware that some people may be allergic to certain essential oils

Dietary Approaches

Diet can play a significant role in managing eczema for some individuals. While there's no one-size-fits-all eczema diet, certain dietary approaches may help reduce inflammation and improve symptoms.

1. Anti-Inflammatory Diet:
   - Focus on foods rich in omega-3 fatty acids (e.g., fatty fish, flaxseeds, chia seeds)
   - Include plenty of fruits and vegetables, particularly those high in antioxidants
   - Limit processed foods, sugar, and unhealthy fats

2. Elimination Diets:
   - Involves removing potential trigger foods and gradually reintroducing them to identify sensitivities
   - Common foods eliminated include dairy, eggs, soy, wheat, peanuts, and tree nuts
   - Should be done under the guidance of a healthcare provider or registered

dietitian

3. Probiotics and Prebiotics:
   - May help balance the gut microbiome, which can influence skin health
   - Some studies suggest probiotics may help reduce eczema severity, particularly in children
   - Can be consumed through fermented foods or supplements

4. Vitamin D:
   - Some studies suggest vitamin D supplementation may help improve eczema symptoms
   - Can be obtained through sunlight exposure, certain foods, or supplements

5. Zinc:
   - Important for skin healing and immune function
   - Some studies suggest zinc supplementation may help improve eczema symptoms
   - Can be found in foods like oysters, beef, pumpkin seeds, or taken as a supplement

6. Quercetin:
   - A flavonoid with anti-inflammatory properties
   - Found in foods like apples, berries, and leafy greens
   - Some preliminary research suggests it may help with eczema symptoms

Remember, dietary changes should be made in consultation with a healthcare provider or registered dietitian to ensure nutritional needs are met, especially for children.

Mind-Body Techniques

Stress is a known trigger for eczema flares, and mind-body techniques can be valuable tools for stress management and overall well-being.

1. Meditation:
   - Can help reduce stress and improve overall well-being
   - Mindfulness meditation may help individuals cope better with eczema symptoms

2. Yoga:
   - Combines physical postures, breathing techniques, and meditation
   - May help reduce stress and improve overall health
   - Some poses may help improve circulation to the skin

3. Progressive Muscle Relaxation:
   - Involves tensing and relaxing different muscle groups
   - Can help reduce stress and may improve sleep quality

4. Biofeedback:
   - Uses sensors to provide information about bodily processes
   - May help individuals learn to control stress responses

5. Hypnosis:
   - Some studies suggest hypnosis may help reduce itching and improve eczema symptoms
   - Should be performed by a trained professional

6. Cognitive Behavioral Therapy (CBT):
   - Can help individuals manage stress and change negative thought patterns
   - May be particularly helpful for dealing with the psychological impact of eczema

These techniques can be valuable additions to an eczema management plan, helping to reduce stress and improve overall quality of life.

Acupuncture and Traditional Chinese Medicine

Acupuncture and Traditional Chinese Medicine (TCM) have been used for centuries to treat various conditions, including skin disorders.

1. Acupuncture:
   - Involves inserting thin needles into specific points on the body
   - Some studies suggest it may help reduce itching and improve eczema symptoms
   - Mechanism not fully understood, but may involve modulation of the immune system

2. Chinese Herbal Medicine:
   - Often used in combination with acupuncture
   - Some formulations have shown promise in clinical trials for eczema
   - Caution is needed as some preparations may contain steroids or other undisclosed ingredients

3. Moxibustion:
   - Involves burning mugwort herb near acupuncture points
   - Sometimes used in conjunction with acupuncture for eczema treatment

When considering TCM:
   - Seek treatment from a licensed practitioner
   - Inform your regular healthcare provider about any TCM treatments
   - Be cautious with herbal preparations, as quality and content can vary

Balneotherapy and Climatotherapy

These therapies involve using natural resources for healing.

1. Balneotherapy:
   - Involves bathing in mineral-rich waters
   - Some studies suggest it may help improve skin hydration and reduce inflammation

- Often combined with other treatments at specialized clinics

2. Climatotherapy:
   - Involves traveling to specific climates believed to be beneficial for skin conditions
   - Examples include the Dead Sea region, known for its unique climate and mineral-rich waters
   - May provide temporary relief, but effects often diminish upon returning home

While these therapies can be helpful for some, they may not be practical or accessible for everyone.

Topical Natural Remedies

Various natural substances are sometimes used topically for eczema management:

1. Coconut Oil:
   - Has moisturizing and antimicrobial properties
   - May help improve skin hydration and reduce staph bacteria on the skin

2. Sunflower Seed Oil:
   - Rich in linoleic acid, which may help improve the skin barrier
   - Some studies suggest it may help reduce inflammation and improve skin hydration

3. Honey, particularly Manuka Honey:
   - Has antimicrobial and wound-healing properties
   - May help soothe and moisturize the skin

4. Oatmeal:
   - Has anti-inflammatory and soothing properties

- Can be used in baths or as a paste for spot treatment

5. Apple Cider Vinegar:
  - May help balance skin pH
  - Should be diluted before use and avoided on open wounds

6. Shea Butter:
  - Rich in fatty acids and vitamins
  - May help moisturize and soothe the skin

When using these remedies:
  - Always patch test before widespread use
  - Be aware that natural doesn't always mean safe – allergic reactions can occur
  - These should complement, not replace, your regular eczema care routine

Phototherapy and Light-Based Therapies

While conventional phototherapy is typically administered in a medical setting, some alternative light-based therapies are used for eczema:

1. Red Light Therapy:
  - Uses low-level red or near-infrared light
  - Some preliminary research suggests it may help reduce inflammation and promote healing

2. Blue Light Therapy:
  - May have antimicrobial effects
  - Some studies suggest it might help reduce eczema symptoms

3. Salt Lamps:
  - Claimed to purify air and reduce allergies, though scientific evidence is lacking

- May provide a calming ambiance, which could indirectly help with stress-related flares

While some of these therapies show promise, more research is needed to establish their efficacy and safety for eczema treatment.

Lifestyle Modifications

In addition to specific therapies, certain lifestyle modifications can complement eczema management:

1. Clothing Choices:
   - Wear soft, breathable fabrics like cotton
   - Avoid wool and synthetic fibers that can irritate the skin

2. Temperature Control:
   - Maintain a cool, consistent temperature in living spaces
   - Avoid overheating during sleep or exercise

3. Humidity Management:
   - Use a humidifier in dry environments to add moisture to the air

4. Gentle Exercise:
   - Regular, gentle exercise can help reduce stress and improve overall health
   - Be mindful of sweat management during workouts

5. Stress Reduction Techniques:
   - Practice stress management techniques like deep breathing or journaling

6. Sleep Hygiene:
   - Prioritize good sleep habits, as poor sleep can exacerbate eczema symptoms

7. Avoiding Triggers:
   - Identify and avoid personal eczema triggers, which may include certain foods, environmental factors, or stress

These lifestyle modifications can significantly impact eczema management when combined with other treatments.

The Role of Complementary and Alternative Medicine (CAM) in Eczema Management

While many people find relief with natural and alternative therapies, it's important to approach these treatments with a balanced perspective:

Potential Benefits:
   - May provide additional symptom relief
   - Can empower individuals to take an active role in their care
   - Often focus on overall health and well-being, not just symptom management
   - May have fewer side effects than some conventional treatments

Considerations:
   - Scientific evidence is limited for many CAM therapies
   - Natural doesn't always mean safe – side effects and interactions can occur
   - Quality and purity of natural products can vary
   - May be costly and not covered by insurance

Best Practices for Incorporating CAM:

1. Communicate with your healthcare provider about any CAM therapies you're considering or using
2. Don't stop prescribed treatments without consulting your healthcare provider
3. Be wary of claims that seem too good to be true

4. Choose high-quality products from reputable sources
5. Keep a diary to track the effects of any new treatments

Integrative Approach to Eczema Management

An integrative approach to eczema management combines the best of conventional medicine with evidence-based complementary therapies. This approach:
- Considers the whole person, not just the skin condition
- Emphasizes the importance of the patient-provider relationship
- Focuses on lifestyle factors that influence health
- Uses the least invasive, least toxic interventions first
- Remains open to new paradigms of treatment

Conclusion: Expanding the Toolbox for Eczema Management

Natural and alternative therapies can offer valuable additions to the eczema management toolbox. While they shouldn't replace conventional treatments, they can complement them, potentially enhancing overall effectiveness and improving quality of life.

As with any aspect of eczema management, what works best can vary greatly from person to person. Patience, careful observation, and open communication with healthcare providers are key to finding the most effective combination of treatments.

Remember, the goal is not just to manage symptoms, but to promote overall skin health and well-being. By considering a range of approaches – from conventional treatments to natural remedies and lifestyle modifications – individuals with eczema can develop a comprehensive, personalized management plan that addresses their unique needs and preferences.

As research in this area continues to evolve, we may see more integration of natural and alternative therapies into mainstream eczema care. Until then, an open-minded yet critical approach to these therapies, always in consultation with healthcare providers, can help individuals make informed decisions about their eczema management.

CHAPTER 7

The Eczema Diet: Nutrition for Healthy Skin

The relationship between diet and eczema is complex and often individualized. While there's no one-size-fits-all "eczema diet," growing evidence suggests that dietary factors can play a significant role in managing eczema for many individuals. In this chapter, we'll explore how nutrition can impact skin health, discuss foods that may trigger or alleviate eczema symptoms, and provide practical guidance for using diet as part of a comprehensive eczema management strategy.

The Skin-Gut Connection

To understand how diet can influence eczema, it's important to first recognize the intimate connection between gut health and skin health, often referred to as the "gut-skin axis."

Key points:

1. The gut microbiome plays a crucial role in immune function and overall health.
2. Imbalances in the gut microbiome (dysbiosis) have been linked to various skin conditions, including eczema.
3. What we eat directly influences our gut microbiome composition.
4. A healthy gut barrier helps prevent the absorption of allergens and

toxins that could trigger immune responses.

5. Inflammation in the gut can lead to systemic inflammation, potentially exacerbating skin inflammation.

Understanding this connection helps explain why dietary changes can have a significant impact on skin health and eczema symptoms for many individuals.

Foods to Avoid

While individual triggers can vary, certain foods are more commonly associated with eczema flare-ups. It's important to note that not everyone with eczema will react to these foods, and elimination should be done carefully and under professional guidance.

1. Dairy Products:
   - Cow's milk, in particular, is a common trigger for many people with eczema.
   - Casein and whey proteins in milk can be allergenic for some individuals.
   - Consider alternatives like almond milk, oat milk, or coconut milk.

2. Eggs:
   - Both egg whites and yolks can be problematic for some people with eczema.
   - Eggs are often hidden ingredients in many processed foods.

3. Gluten-containing Grains:
   - Wheat, barley, and rye contain gluten, which can trigger symptoms in sensitive individuals.
   - Non-celiac gluten sensitivity may play a role in some cases of eczema.

4. Soy:
   - Soy is a common allergen and may trigger eczema symptoms in some

people.
   - It's often used as an additive in many processed foods.

5. Nuts:
   - Tree nuts and peanuts are common allergens that may exacerbate eczema in sensitive individuals.
   - Even if not allergic, some people find nuts inflammatory.

6. Citrus Fruits:
   - While rich in vitamin C, citrus fruits can be acidic and may irritate sensitive skin.
   - Some people report increased itching after consuming citrus.

7. Tomatoes:
   - Part of the nightshade family, tomatoes may trigger inflammation in some individuals.
   - Other nightshades to watch include potatoes, peppers, and eggplants.

8. Processed Foods:
   - High in additives, preservatives, and artificial ingredients that may trigger reactions.
   - Often contain hidden allergens and inflammatory ingredients.

9. Refined Sugars:
   - Can contribute to inflammation in the body.
   - May feed harmful gut bacteria, potentially disrupting the gut-skin axis.

10. Alcohol:
   - Can be dehydrating and may worsen skin dryness.
   - Some people report increased itching after alcohol consumption.

It's crucial to remember that these are general guidelines. Not everyone with eczema will need to avoid all these foods, and some may have unique triggers not listed here. Keeping a food diary and working with a healthcare provider or registered dietitian can help identify individual triggers.

Beneficial Foods for Eczema

While avoiding trigger foods is important, focusing on nutrient-rich, anti-inflammatory foods can also play a crucial role in managing eczema.

1. Fatty Fish:
    - Rich in omega-3 fatty acids, which have anti-inflammatory properties.
    - Examples include salmon, mackerel, sardines, and herring.
    - Aim for 2-3 servings per week.

2. Probiotic-Rich Foods:
    - Help support a healthy gut microbiome.
    - Include yogurt (if dairy is tolerated), kefir, sauerkraut, kimchi, and kombucha.

3. Prebiotic Foods:
    - Feed beneficial gut bacteria.
    - Include garlic, onions, leeks, asparagus, and bananas.

4. Quercetin-Rich Foods:
    - Quercetin is a flavonoid with anti-inflammatory and antihistamine properties.
    - Found in apples, berries, broccoli, kale, and onions.

5. Vitamin D-Rich Foods:
    - Vitamin D deficiency has been linked to increased eczema severity.
    - Include fatty fish, egg yolks (if tolerated), and fortified foods.

6. Zinc-Rich Foods:
    - Zinc is important for skin healing and immune function.

- Include oysters, beef, pumpkin seeds, and lentils.

7. Antioxidant-Rich Foods:
   - Help combat oxidative stress and inflammation.
   - Include a variety of colorful fruits and vegetables, especially berries, leafy greens, and sweet potatoes.

8. Collagen-Boosting Foods:
   - Support skin health and healing.
   - Include bone broth, chicken, fish, and foods high in vitamin C like bell peppers and strawberries.

9. Anti-Inflammatory Herbs and Spices:
   - Turmeric, ginger, cinnamon, and garlic have potent anti-inflammatory properties.
   - Can be incorporated into cooking or taken as supplements (under professional guidance).

10. Green Tea:
   - Rich in polyphenols with anti-inflammatory properties.
   - May help reduce oxidative stress in the body.

Incorporating these foods into your diet can support overall skin health and potentially help manage eczema symptoms. However, it's important to introduce new foods gradually and monitor for any reactions.

The Role of Specific Nutrients

Certain nutrients play key roles in skin health and immune function. Ensuring adequate intake of these nutrients can support overall skin health and potentially help manage eczema:

1. Omega-3 Fatty Acids:

- Have anti-inflammatory properties.
- Help maintain skin barrier function.
- Sources: fatty fish, flaxseeds, chia seeds, walnuts.

2. Vitamin D:
   - Important for immune function and skin barrier health.
   - Deficiency is common in people with eczema.
   - Sources: sunlight exposure, fatty fish, fortified foods, supplements.

3. Vitamin E:
   - Antioxidant that supports skin health.
   - May help reduce inflammation and support skin barrier function.
   - Sources: nuts, seeds, avocados, leafy greens.

4. Zinc:
   - Important for skin healing and immune function.
   - Sources: oysters, beef, pumpkin seeds, lentils.

5. Vitamin C:
   - Antioxidant that supports collagen production and skin healing.
   - Sources: citrus fruits (if tolerated), bell peppers, strawberries, broccoli.

6. B Vitamins:
   - Important for skin health and overall cellular function.
   - Sources: whole grains, legumes, nuts, seeds, leafy greens.

7. Selenium:
   - Antioxidant that supports immune function.
   - Sources: Brazil nuts, fish, whole grains.

8. Flavonoids:
   - Plant compounds with anti-inflammatory and antioxidant properties.
   - Sources: berries, citrus fruits, tea, dark chocolate.

While a balanced diet should provide most of these nutrients, in some cases, supplementation may be recommended under healthcare provider guidance.

Hydration and Eczema

Proper hydration is crucial for skin health and can play a significant role in managing eczema:

1. Water:
   - Helps maintain skin hydration from the inside out.
   - Aim for at least 8 glasses of water per day, more if active or in hot weather.

2. Herbal Teas:
   - Can contribute to hydration while providing additional benefits.
   - Chamomile and green tea may have anti-inflammatory properties.

3. Hydrating Foods:
   - Foods with high water content can contribute to hydration.
   - Include cucumbers, watermelon, zucchini, and celery.

4. Limiting Dehydrating Substances:
   - Reduce intake of caffeine and alcohol, which can be dehydrating.

Remember, while topical moisturizing is crucial, internal hydration is equally important for maintaining skin health.

Elimination Diets and Food Challenges

For some individuals with eczema, identifying and eliminating specific food triggers can significantly improve symptoms. An elimination diet followed by controlled food challenges is often the most effective way to identify these triggers.

Steps in an elimination diet:

1. Remove suspected trigger foods from the diet for a set period (usually 2-4 weeks).
2. Monitor symptoms for improvement.
3. Gradually reintroduce eliminated foods one at a time, monitoring for reactions.
4. If a reaction occurs, that food is identified as a potential trigger and may need to be avoided long-term.

Common foods eliminated include:
- Dairy
- Eggs
- Soy
- Wheat/gluten
- Nuts
- Fish/shellfish

Important considerations:
- Elimination diets should be done under the guidance of a healthcare provider or registered dietitian to ensure nutritional needs are met.
- They can be challenging and may not be appropriate for everyone, especially children.
- Not all food reactions are immediate; some can occur up to 48 hours after consumption.

Meal Planning and Recipes

Implementing dietary changes for eczema management can be challenging. Here are some tips and ideas to help:

1. Plan Ahead:

- Meal planning can help ensure a balanced diet while avoiding trigger foods.
   - Prepare batches of safe foods in advance for busy days.

2. Read Labels Carefully:
   - Many packaged foods contain hidden allergens or inflammatory ingredients.
   - Look for products specifically labeled as free from your trigger foods.

3. Focus on Whole Foods:
   - Build meals around fresh fruits, vegetables, lean proteins, and safe grains.
   - Minimize processed foods to reduce exposure to additives and preservatives.

4. Experiment with Alternatives:
   - Try dairy-free milks like almond or oat milk.
   - Explore gluten-free grains like quinoa, rice, and buckwheat.
   - Use plant-based proteins like lentils and chickpeas if animal proteins are problematic.

5. Make Your Own:
   - Prepare homemade versions of foods to control ingredients.
   - Make your own salad dressings, sauces, and snacks to avoid hidden triggers.

Sample Meal Ideas:

Breakfast:
   - Oatmeal (if tolerated) with berries, chia seeds, and a dollop of coconut yogurt
   - Smoothie bowl with spinach, banana, avocado, and seed butter

Lunch:

- Grilled chicken salad with mixed greens, avocado, and olive oil dressing
- Lentil soup with carrots, celery, and turmeric

Dinner:
- Baked salmon with roasted sweet potato and steamed broccoli
- Quinoa stir-fry with mixed vegetables and tofu (if tolerated)

Snacks:
- Apple slices with seed butter
- Homemade trail mix with safe nuts/seeds and dried fruit
- Vegetable sticks with homemade hummus

Remember to adjust these ideas based on your individual tolerances and triggers.

Nutritional Supplements for Eczema

While a balanced diet should be the primary focus, certain supplements may be beneficial for some individuals with eczema. Always consult with a healthcare provider before starting any supplement regimen.

1. Probiotics:
   - May help balance the gut microbiome and modulate immune function.
   - Look for strains specifically studied for eczema, such as Lactobacillus rhamnosus GG.

2. Omega-3 Fatty Acids:
   - Fish oil or algae-based supplements can provide anti-inflammatory benefits.
   - Dosage should be determined by a healthcare provider.

3. Vitamin D:
   - Supplementation may be recommended if blood levels are low.

- Dosage should be based on individual needs and current levels.

4. Evening Primrose Oil:
   - Contains gamma-linolenic acid (GLA), which may help with skin barrier function.
   - Evidence is mixed, but some individuals find it helpful.

5. Zinc:
   - May be beneficial if deficient, but over-supplementation can be harmful.
   - Blood tests can determine if supplementation is needed.

6. Vitamin E:
   - Antioxidant properties may support skin health.
   - Can be applied topically or taken orally.

7. Collagen:
   - May support skin healing and overall skin health.
   - Available in powder or capsule form.

Remember, supplements are not regulated as strictly as medications. Choose high-quality products from reputable sources and always inform your healthcare provider about any supplements you're taking.

Special Considerations for Children

Dietary management of eczema in children requires special care:

1. Balanced Nutrition:
   - Ensure that elimination diets don't compromise overall nutrition and growth.
   - Work with a pediatric dietitian to ensure nutritional needs are met.

2. Gradual Introduction:

- Introduce new foods one at a time to easily identify any reactions.
- Follow current guidelines for introducing potential allergens to infants.

3. Breastfeeding:
   - If breastfeeding, the mother's diet may influence the baby's eczema.
   - Maternal elimination diets should be done under professional guidance.

4. Formula Considerations:
   - For infants with cow's milk allergy, hypoallergenic formulas may be recommended.
   - Soy-based formulas may not be suitable as soy is also a common allergen.

5. Supplements:
   - Dosages for children differ from adults and should be carefully determined by a healthcare provider.

6. Family Approach:
   - Involve the whole family in dietary changes to support the child with eczema.
   - Make healthy eating a positive, inclusive experience.

Monitoring and Adjusting Your Eczema Diet

Managing eczema through diet is often a process of trial and error. Here are some tips for monitoring progress and making adjustments:

1. Keep a Food and Symptom Diary:
   - Record everything you eat and drink, along with any eczema symptoms.
   - Look for patterns over time.

2. Be Patient:
   - Dietary changes can take weeks to show effects on the skin.
   - Give each change at least 2-4 weeks before evaluating its impact.

3. Consider Other Factors:
   - Remember that diet is just one aspect of eczema management.
   - Consider other triggers like stress, weather, and skincare products.

4. Regular Check-ins:
   - Have regular follow-ups with your healthcare provider or dietitian.
   - Discuss any concerns or difficulties with maintaining the diet.

5. Reintroduction Tests:
   - Periodically retest eliminated foods to see if tolerances have changed.
   - This is especially important for children, as food allergies can sometimes be outgrown.

6. Adjust as Needed:
   - Be prepared to modify your diet as your eczema changes or as you discover new triggers or safe foods.

7. Nutritional Balance:
   - Regularly assess your diet to ensure you're meeting all nutritional needs.
   - Consider working with a registered dietitian for ongoing support.

Conclusion: Nourishing Your Skin from Within

Diet can play a significant role in managing eczema, but it's important to approach dietary changes as part of a comprehensive management plan. What works for one person may not work for another, and finding the right balance often requires patience and persistence.

Remember these key points:
   - There's no one-size-fits-all eczema diet.
   - Focus on whole, nutrient-dense foods that support overall health.
   - Work with healthcare providers to ensure nutritional needs are met, especially when eliminating foods.

- Be patient and consistent in your approach.
- Combine dietary strategies with other eczema management techniques for best results.

By nourishing your body with the right foods and avoiding personal triggers, you can support your skin's health from the inside out. While diet alone may not cure eczema, for many people, it can be a powerful tool in managing symptoms and improving overall quality of life.

As research in this area continues to evolve, we may gain even more insights into the relationship between diet and eczema. Stay informed, work closely with your healthcare team, and remember that you are your own best advocate in finding the dietary approach that works best for your eczema management.

CHAPTER 8

Lifestyle Modifications for Eczema Management

While medical treatments and dietary approaches play crucial roles in managing eczema, lifestyle modifications can significantly impact the frequency and severity of flare-ups. In this chapter, we'll explore various lifestyle changes and strategies that can help individuals with eczema better manage their condition and improve their overall quality of life.

Stress Reduction Techniques

Stress is a well-known trigger for eczema flares. Managing stress effectively can help reduce the frequency and severity of symptoms.

1. Mindfulness Meditation:
    - Focuses on being present in the moment
    - Can help reduce stress and anxiety
    - Start with short sessions (5-10 minutes) and gradually increase duration
    - Use guided meditation apps or videos for support

2. Deep Breathing Exercises:
    - Activates the body's relaxation response
    - Try the 4-7-8 technique: Inhale for 4 counts, hold for 7, exhale for 8
    - Practice regularly, especially during stressful moments

3. Progressive Muscle Relaxation:
    - Involves tensing and relaxing different muscle groups
    - Can help reduce physical tension associated with stress
    - Particularly useful before bedtime to improve sleep quality

4. Yoga:
    - Combines physical postures, breathing techniques, and meditation
    - Choose gentle forms of yoga to avoid excessive sweating
    - Restorative or yin yoga can be particularly beneficial for stress reduction

5. Regular Exercise:
    - Releases endorphins, which can improve mood and reduce stress
    - Choose low-impact activities like walking, swimming, or cycling
    - Be mindful of sweat management to avoid irritating the skin

6. Journaling:
    - Helps process emotions and identify stress triggers
    - Try gratitude journaling to focus on positive aspects of life
    - Use as a tool to track eczema triggers and patterns

7. Time Management:
    - Poor time management can lead to increased stress
    - Use tools like calendars and to-do lists to stay organized
    - Learn to prioritize tasks and say no to non-essential commitments

8. Cognitive Behavioral Therapy (CBT):
    - A type of therapy that helps change negative thought patterns
    - Can be particularly helpful for dealing with the psychological impact of
eczema
    - Consider working with a therapist trained in CBT

Remember, stress reduction is a skill that improves with practice. Experiment with different techniques to find what works best for you.

Exercise and Physical Activity

Regular exercise is important for overall health and can help manage eczema when done correctly.

Benefits of Exercise for Eczema:
- Reduces stress
- Improves circulation
- Boosts immune function
- Enhances overall well-being

Considerations for Exercising with Eczema:
1. Choose Low-Impact Activities:
- Swimming (in chlorine-free pools if possible)
- Walking
- Yoga
- Tai Chi
- Cycling

2. Manage Sweat:
- Wear moisture-wicking clothing
- Shower and moisturize immediately after exercise
- Use a soft towel to pat skin dry, don't rub

3. Stay Hydrated:
- Drink plenty of water before, during, and after exercise
- Proper hydration helps maintain skin moisture

4. Time Your Workouts:
- Exercise in cooler parts of the day to minimize sweating
- Avoid outdoor workouts during high pollen times if you have allergies

5. Protect Your Skin:

- Use breathable, loose-fitting workout clothes
- Apply moisturizer before exercising to create a barrier

6. Listen to Your Body:
  - If a particular activity irritates your skin, try alternatives
  - Take rest days when needed, especially during flare-ups

Remember, the goal is to find a balance between staying active and managing your eczema symptoms.

Sleep Hygiene and Eczema

Quality sleep is crucial for overall health and can significantly impact eczema symptoms. Poor sleep can increase stress and inflammation, potentially exacerbating eczema.

Tips for Better Sleep with Eczema:
  1. Maintain a Consistent Sleep Schedule:
  - Go to bed and wake up at the same time every day, even on weekends
  - This helps regulate your body's internal clock

2. Create a Relaxing Bedtime Routine:
  - Engage in calming activities before bed (reading, gentle stretching, listening to soothing music)
  - Avoid screens for at least an hour before bedtime due to blue light exposure

3. Optimize Your Sleep Environment:
  - Keep your bedroom cool (around 65°F or 18°C)
  - Use a humidifier to add moisture to the air
  - Ensure your room is dark and quiet

4. Choose Eczema-Friendly Bedding:

- Use natural, breathable fabrics like 100% cotton
- Wash bedding weekly in fragrance-free, hypoallergenic detergent
- Consider using dust mite-proof covers on pillows and mattresses

5. Manage Nighttime Itching:
  - Apply moisturizer before bed
  - Keep fingernails short and consider wearing cotton gloves to prevent scratching
  - Use cool compresses if itching is severe

6. Be Mindful of Evening Habits:
  - Avoid caffeine and alcohol in the hours before bedtime
  - Don't eat heavy meals close to bedtime

7. Consider Sleep Positioning:
  - Elevate your head slightly to reduce facial swelling if you have facial eczema
  - Use pillows to prevent skin-on-skin contact in problem areas

If sleep problems persist, consult with your healthcare provider. They may recommend additional strategies or treatments to improve your sleep quality.

Clothing and Fabric Choices

The clothes you wear can have a significant impact on your eczema. Choosing the right fabrics and styles can help reduce irritation and manage symptoms.

Best Fabrics for Eczema-Prone Skin:
  1. Cotton:
  - Soft, natural, and breathable
  - Allows skin to breathe and helps regulate body temperature

2. Silk:

- Smooth and cool to the touch
- Can be beneficial for some people with eczema, especially for bedding

3. Bamboo:
   - Soft, moisture-wicking, and naturally antimicrobial
   - Good option for workout clothes

4. TENCEL™ (Lyocell):
   - Made from wood pulp, soft and breathable
   - Effective at moisture management

Fabrics to Avoid:
   1. Wool:
   - Can be itchy and irritating for many people with eczema

2. Synthetic Fabrics:
   - Polyester, nylon, and other synthetics can trap heat and moisture

3. Rough Fabrics:
   - Denim, canvas, and other rough materials can irritate the skin

Clothing Tips for Eczema Management:
   1. Choose Loose-Fitting Clothes:
   - Allows air circulation and reduces friction

2. Remove Labels:
   - Cut out scratchy labels from clothes

3. Wear Layers:
   - Allows for easy adjustment to temperature changes

4. Be Mindful of Seams:
   - Look for clothes with flat seams or wear them inside out to reduce

irritation

5. Consider Special Eczema Clothing:
   - Some brands make clothes specifically designed for eczema-prone skin

6. Wash New Clothes Before Wearing:
   - Removes potential irritants from the manufacturing process

Remember to choose clothes that not only manage your eczema but also make you feel comfortable and confident.

Environmental Controls

Your environment can significantly impact your eczema. Making certain changes at home and in your daily surroundings can help reduce triggers and manage symptoms.

1. Temperature and Humidity Control:
   - Maintain a consistent, cool temperature in your home
   - Use a humidifier to keep humidity levels between 30-50%
   - Avoid sudden temperature changes when possible

2. Dust Control:
   - Use dust mite-proof covers on pillows and mattresses
   - Vacuum regularly using a HEPA filter vacuum
   - Reduce clutter to minimize dust accumulation

3. Air Quality:
   - Use an air purifier with a HEPA filter
   - Keep windows closed during high pollen days if you have allergies
   - Avoid smoking and secondhand smoke

4. Cleaning Products:

- Use fragrance-free, hypoallergenic cleaning products
- Consider natural cleaning alternatives like vinegar and baking soda
- Wear gloves when cleaning to protect your hands

5. Laundry:
   - Use fragrance-free, hypoallergenic laundry detergent
   - Double rinse clothes to remove all detergent residue
   - Avoid fabric softeners and dryer sheets

6. Pet Management:
   - Keep pets out of the bedroom if you're allergic
   - Bathe pets regularly to reduce dander
   - Vacuum frequently in homes with pets

7. Water Quality:
   - Consider using a water softener if you live in a hard water area
   - Use a shower filter to remove chlorine and other potential irritants

8. Outdoor Considerations:
   - Check pollen forecasts and plan outdoor activities accordingly
   - Shower and change clothes after spending time outdoors during high pollen seasons

By controlling your environment, you can significantly reduce exposure to potential eczema triggers.

Stress Management in Daily Life

While we've discussed specific stress reduction techniques, managing stress in your daily life is crucial for long-term eczema control.

1. Identify Stress Triggers:
   - Keep a stress diary to identify patterns and common stressors

   - Once identified, develop strategies to address or avoid these triggers

2. Practice Time Management:
   - Use calendars and to-do lists to stay organized
   - Break large tasks into smaller, manageable steps
   - Learn to prioritize and say no to non-essential commitments

3. Establish Boundaries:
   - Learn to set healthy boundaries in personal and professional relationships
   - Communicate your needs clearly and respectfully

4. Cultivate Supportive Relationships:
   - Surround yourself with positive, supportive people
   - Don't hesitate to seek help when needed

5. Develop Healthy Coping Mechanisms:
   - Find healthy ways to deal with stress (e.g., exercise, hobbies, creative activities)
   - Avoid unhealthy coping mechanisms like excessive alcohol consumption or emotional eating

6. Practice Self-Care:
   - Make time for activities you enjoy
   - Prioritize sleep and regular meals
   - Maintain a consistent skincare routine

7. Consider Professional Help:
   - If stress feels overwhelming, consider talking to a therapist or counselor
   - They can provide additional tools and strategies for stress management

Remember, managing stress is an ongoing process. Be patient with yourself and celebrate small victories in your stress management journey.

Occupational Considerations

For many people with eczema, work environments can present unique challenges. Here are some strategies to manage eczema in the workplace:

1. Communicate with Your Employer:
   - Inform your employer about your condition and any necessary accommodations
   - Many employers are willing to make reasonable adjustments to support employees with chronic conditions

2. Protect Your Hands:
   - Use protective gloves for tasks that involve water or irritants
   - Consider cotton glove liners to absorb sweat
   - Keep moisturizer accessible for frequent application

3. Manage Workplace Stress:
   - Take regular breaks to reduce stress
   - Practice stress-reduction techniques during the workday (e.g., deep breathing, short meditation sessions)

4. Adjust Your Workspace:
   - If possible, sit away from air vents or windows to avoid temperature fluctuations
   - Use a small humidifier at your desk if the air is dry

5. Choose Work-Appropriate Clothing:
   - Opt for breathable, natural fabrics
   - Layer clothing to adjust to temperature changes

6. Be Prepared:
   - Keep a "rescue kit" with moisturizer, medication, and any other necessary items

7. Consider Your Career Choice:
   - If your eczema is severe, you may need to consider how your career choice impacts your skin
   - Some professions (e.g., hairdressing, healthcare) involve frequent hand washing or exposure to irritants

Remember, many countries have laws protecting individuals with chronic conditions in the workplace. Don't hesitate to advocate for your needs.

Social and Relationship Considerations

Eczema can impact social interactions and relationships. Here are some strategies to navigate these challenges:

1. Educate Others:
   - Help friends, family, and colleagues understand your condition
   - Explain that eczema is not contagious and how it affects your daily life

2. Be Open About Your Needs:
   - Communicate clearly about your triggers and limitations
   - Don't be afraid to speak up if a situation is uncomfortable for your skin

3. Plan Social Activities Mindfully:
   - Choose activities that won't exacerbate your eczema (e.g., avoid hot, sweaty environments if that's a trigger)
   - Have a backup plan in case of unexpected flare-ups

4. Develop Confidence:
   - Remember that your worth is not determined by your skin
   - Consider joining support groups to connect with others who understand your experiences

5. Navigate Intimate Relationships:

- Be open with partners about your condition
- Discuss how eczema might impact physical intimacy and find ways to work around it

6. Manage Social Anxiety:
   - If eczema is causing social anxiety, consider talking to a therapist
   - Practice positive self-talk and challenge negative thoughts about your appearance

7. Advocate for Yourself:
   - Don't hesitate to ask for accommodations when needed
   - Remember, most people will be understanding if you explain your situation

Building a strong support network can make a significant difference in living with eczema. Surround yourself with understanding and supportive people.

Travel and Eczema Management

Traveling with eczema requires some extra planning, but it shouldn't prevent you from exploring the world. Here are some tips for managing eczema while traveling:

1. Pack Smart:
   - Bring all necessary medications and skincare products in your carry-on
   - Pack enough supplies for your entire trip, plus extra in case of delays

2. Research Your Destination:
   - Check the climate and potential environmental triggers at your destination
   - Locate nearby pharmacies or healthcare providers in case of emergencies

3. Prepare for Different Water Types:

- Consider bringing a portable shower filter for hard water areas
- Use bottled water for skincare if tap water irritates your skin

4. Manage Air Travel:
   - Apply extra moisturizer before and during flights due to dry cabin air
   - Stay hydrated during the flight

5. Choose Accommodation Wisely:
   - Look for hotels with allergy-friendly rooms if possible
   - Bring your own pillowcase or sleep sack if bedding is a concern

6. Adapt Your Routine:
   - Try to maintain your skincare routine as much as possible
   - Be flexible and adjust as needed based on climate and activities

7. Plan Your Activities:
   - Balance active days with rest days to avoid overexertion
   - Be mindful of activities that might trigger flare-ups (e.g., swimming in chlorinated pools)

8. Communicate Your Needs:
   - Inform travel companions about your condition and any necessary accommodations
   - Don't hesitate to speak up if a situation is uncomfortable for your skin

With proper planning, you can enjoy traveling while managing your eczema effectively.

Conclusion: Empowerment Through Lifestyle Management

Managing eczema goes beyond medical treatments and skincare routines. By making thoughtful lifestyle modifications, you can significantly impact your eczema symptoms and overall quality of life.

Remember these key points:
- Stress management is crucial for eczema control
- Regular exercise, when done correctly, can benefit your skin and overall health
- Quality sleep is essential for skin health and eczema management
- Your environment, including clothing choices and home conditions, can significantly impact your eczema
- Occupational and social considerations are important aspects of living with eczema
- With proper planning, eczema shouldn't limit your ability to travel and enjoy life

Implementing these lifestyle modifications may take time and effort, but the potential benefits are substantial. Not only can these changes help manage your eczema symptoms, but they can also contribute to better overall health and well-being.

Every person with eczema is unique, and what works best will vary from individual to individual. Be patient with yourself as you explore different strategies, and don't hesitate to adjust your approach as needed. Remember, managing eczema is a journey, not a destination.

By taking control of your lifestyle factors, you're not just managing your eczema – you're empowering yourself to live your best life despite the challenges of this chronic condition. With persistence, self-compassion, and the support of your healthcare team and loved ones, you can develop a lifestyle that supports your skin health and overall well-being.

CHAPTER 9

Skincare Routines and Product Selection

A consistent and appropriate skincare routine is fundamental to managing eczema effectively. In this chapter, we'll explore the key components of an eczema-friendly skincare regimen, discuss how to choose the right products, and provide guidance on establishing a routine that works for you.

The Importance of a Skincare Routine

For individuals with eczema, a tailored skincare routine is not just about beauty—it's a crucial part of managing the condition. A good skincare routine can:

1. Maintain skin hydration
2. Strengthen the skin barrier
3. Reduce inflammation and itching
4. Help prevent flare-ups
5. Enhance the effectiveness of medical treatments

Remember, consistency is key. Even when your skin is clear, maintaining your skincare routine can help prevent future flare-ups.

The Basic Steps of an Eczema Skincare Routine

While individual needs may vary, a basic eczema skincare routine typically includes the following steps:

1. Cleansing
2. Moisturizing
3. Treating (applying medicated products as prescribed)
4. Protecting (from sun and environmental factors)

Let's explore each of these steps in detail.

1. Gentle Cleansing Techniques

Proper cleansing is crucial for removing irritants, allergens, and bacteria from the skin without stripping away natural oils.

Key points for cleansing:

a) Choose the Right Cleanser:
   - Opt for mild, fragrance-free, soap-free cleansers
   - Look for products specifically formulated for sensitive or eczema-prone skin
   - Avoid harsh soaps, which can disrupt the skin's natural pH

b) Water Temperature:
   - Use lukewarm water, not hot
   - Hot water can strip the skin of its natural oils and trigger itching

c) Gentle Techniques:
   - Use your hands or a soft cloth to cleanse

- Avoid scrubbing or using rough washcloths or sponges
- Pat or dab the skin, don't rub

d) Frequency:
  - Cleanse once or twice daily, or as recommended by your dermatologist
  - Over-cleansing can dry out the skin

e) Special Considerations:
  - For facial eczema, consider the oil cleansing method or micellar water
  - For hand eczema, use gentle hand washes and always moisturize after washing

Remember, the goal of cleansing is to remove impurities without compromising the skin barrier.

2. Moisturizing Strategies

Moisturizing is perhaps the most critical step in an eczema skincare routine. It helps hydrate the skin, repair the skin barrier, and lock in moisture.

Key points for moisturizing:

a) Choose the Right Moisturizer:
  - Look for products with ingredients like ceramides, hyaluronic acid, and glycerin
  - Ointments are most effective for very dry skin, followed by creams, then lotions
  - Avoid products with potential irritants like fragrances, dyes, or certain preservatives

b) Timing:
  - Apply moisturizer immediately after bathing or washing, while the skin is still damp

- This helps lock in moisture

c) Frequency:
   - Moisturize at least twice daily, or more often if needed
   - Pay extra attention to problem areas

d) Application Technique:
   - Apply moisturizer in a downward motion, following the direction of hair growth
   - Be gentle – don't rub or pull at the skin

e) Quantity:
   - Use generous amounts – most people under-apply moisturizer
   - A good rule of thumb is to use enough that the skin feels slippery, not sticky

f) Consider Occlusion:
   - For very dry areas, consider applying moisturizer and then covering with a damp cloth or plastic wrap for a short period
   - This technique, known as occlusion, can significantly increase hydration

Remember, finding the right moisturizer may take some trial and error. What works for one person may not work for another.

3. Treating: Applying Medicated Products

If your healthcare provider has prescribed topical medications, it's important to use them correctly as part of your skincare routine.

Key points for treatment application:

a) Follow Prescriptions:
   - Use medications exactly as prescribed

- Don't stop using a medication without consulting your healthcare provider, even if symptoms improve

b) Order of Application:
   - Generally, apply medications to clean, dry skin before moisturizer
   - Wait a few minutes between applying medication and moisturizer

c) Use the Right Amount:
   - For topical corticosteroids, use the fingertip unit (FTU) method to ensure you're using the correct amount

d) Be Aware of Side Effects:
   - Know the potential side effects of your medications and report any concerns to your healthcare provider

e) Consider the Sandwich Method:
   - For very dry skin, some dermatologists recommend applying a light layer of moisturizer, then medication, then another layer of moisturizer

Always consult your healthcare provider about how to incorporate prescribed treatments into your skincare routine.

4. Protecting: Sun Protection and Environmental Defense

Protecting your skin from the sun and other environmental factors is crucial for managing eczema.

Key points for protection:

a) Sun Protection:
   - Use a broad-spectrum, hypoallergenic sunscreen with at least SPF 30
   - Look for mineral-based sunscreens (zinc oxide or titanium dioxide) as they're less likely to irritate

- Apply sunscreen as the last step in your morning skincare routine

b) Protective Clothing:
  - Wear loose-fitting, breathable clothing to protect your skin
  - Consider UPF (Ultraviolet Protection Factor) clothing for extra sun protection

c) Environmental Defense:
  - Use a humidifier in dry environments
  - Avoid extreme temperature changes when possible
  - Protect your skin from harsh winds with appropriate clothing

d) Avoid Triggers:
  - Identify and avoid environmental triggers like certain fabrics, dust, or pet dander

Remember, protection is about both what you put on your skin and how you manage your environment.

Choosing Eczema-Friendly Products

Selecting the right skincare products is crucial for managing eczema. Here are some guidelines:

1. Read Labels Carefully:
  - Look for products labeled "fragrance-free" (not just "unscented")
  - Avoid common irritants like alcohol, retinoids, and alpha-hydroxy acids
  - Be cautious with "natural" products – natural doesn't always mean skin-friendly

2. Consider Ingredients:
  - Beneficial ingredients include ceramides, hyaluronic acid, glycerin, and niacinamide

- Avoid products with known irritants like fragrances, essential oils, and harsh preservatives

3. Choose the Right Formulation:
    - For very dry skin, ointments are most effective
    - Creams are good for normal to dry skin
    - Lotions are lightest and good for less dry areas or in hot, humid weather

4. Patch Test:
    - Always patch test new products on a small area of skin for at least 48 hours before widespread use

5. Simplify Your Routine:
    - Use fewer products with minimal ingredients
    - Avoid trendy multi-step routines that can overwhelm sensitive skin

6. Consider Your Skin Type:
    - Eczema can occur with any skin type – oily, dry, or combination
    - Choose products that address both your eczema and your overall skin type

7. Look for Certified Products:
    - Some organizations certify products as eczema-friendly
    - While not a guarantee, these can be a helpful starting point

Remember, what works for one person may not work for another. Be patient and prepared to try different products to find what works best for you.

Establishing Your Routine

Creating a skincare routine that works for you is a personal process. Here are some tips:

1. Start Simple:
   - Begin with just the basics: a gentle cleanser, moisturizer, and sunscreen
   - Add additional products slowly, one at a time

2. Be Consistent:
   - Try to perform your routine at the same times each day
   - Consistency helps you establish a habit and allows you to better evaluate what's working

3. Listen to Your Skin:
   - Pay attention to how your skin reacts to different products and environmental factors
   - Keep a skin diary to track changes and identify patterns

4. Adjust as Needed:
   - Be prepared to modify your routine based on:
   - Seasonal changes
   - Stress levels
   - Hormonal fluctuations
   - Flare-ups

5. Don't Overdo It:
   - More is not always better when it comes to skincare
   - Over-cleansing or using too many products can irritate the skin

6. Be Patient:
   - It can take several weeks to see the full effects of a new skincare routine
   - Give new products time to work before deciding if they're effective

7. Consider Your Lifestyle:
   - Your skincare routine should fit into your daily life
   - If a routine is too complicated or time-consuming, you're less likely to stick with it

Sample Eczema Skincare Routines

Here are some sample routines to give you an idea of how to structure your skincare:

Morning Routine:

1. Rinse face with lukewarm water or use a gentle cleanser if needed
2. While skin is damp, apply moisturizer
3. Apply prescribed topical medications (if any)
4. Finish with a mineral-based sunscreen

Evening Routine:

1. Cleanse with a gentle, soap-free cleanser
2. While skin is damp, apply moisturizer
3. Apply prescribed topical medications (if any)
4. For very dry areas, consider applying an occlusive ointment

Additional Considerations:
   - After hand washing: Always apply hand cream
   - Before bed: Consider applying an extra layer of moisturizer or ointment
   - As needed: Reapply moisturizer throughout the day, especially after water exposure

Remember to adjust these routines based on your individual needs and your healthcare provider's recommendations.

Special Considerations for Different Body Areas

Eczema can affect different parts of the body, each requiring slightly different care:

1. Facial Eczema:
    - Use extra-gentle cleansers, potentially micellar water or oil cleansing
    - Choose lighter moisturizers to avoid clogging pores
    - Be cautious with topical medications, as facial skin is more sensitive

2. Hand Eczema:
    - Use lukewarm water and gentle cleansers for washing
    - Apply hand cream after every wash
    - Consider wearing cotton gloves at night after applying thick moisturizer
    - Use protective gloves for household chores

3. Body Eczema:
    - Take short, lukewarm showers or baths
    - Apply moisturizer immediately after bathing
    - Consider using moisturizing body washes instead of soap

4. Scalp Eczema:
    - Use gentle, fragrance-free shampoos
    - Try medicated shampoos if recommended by your healthcare provider
    - Avoid very hot water when washing your hair

5. Eyelid Eczema:
    - Be extremely gentle when cleansing this delicate area
    - Use products specifically tested for use around eyes
    - Consult your healthcare provider, as this area may require special treatment

Addressing Common Skincare Challenges

Even with a good routine, you may encounter some challenges:

1. Persistent Dryness:
   - Try switching to a heavier moisturizer
   - Consider using occlusive ointments at night
   - Ensure you're drinking enough water and using a humidifier

2. Product Reactions:
   - If you suspect a product is causing irritation, stop using it immediately
   - Return to your basic routine until your skin calms down
   - Reintroduce products one at a time to identify the culprit

3. Seasonal Changes:
   - Be prepared to adjust your routine as the seasons change
   - You may need heavier moisturizers in winter and lighter ones in summer

4. Sweating:
   - Rinse off sweat as soon as possible after exercise
   - Change out of damp clothes promptly
   - Consider using moisture-wicking fabrics for workouts

5. Flare-Ups:
   - Have a "rescue routine" ready for flare-ups
   - This might include more frequent moisturizing and use of prescribed medications
   - Avoid any potentially irritating products during flares

6. Itching:
   - Keep moisturizer in the refrigerator for a cooling effect when applied
   - Use cool compresses to soothe itchy skin
   - Consider using itch-relieving products recommended by your healthcare provider

The Role of Non-Topical Treatments in Your Skincare Routine

While this chapter focuses on topical skincare, it's important to remember that other treatments can complement your routine:

1. Oral Medications:
   - If prescribed, take as directed by your healthcare provider
   - Be aware of any skincare precautions associated with your medications

2. Phototherapy:
   - If you're undergoing light therapy, you may need to adjust your skincare routine
   - Always use sun protection as directed by your healthcare provider

3. Stress Management:
   - Incorporate stress-reduction techniques into your daily routine
   - Consider activities like meditation or yoga as part of your overall skin health plan

4. Diet:
   - Stay hydrated
   - Consider incorporating skin-friendly foods into your diet

5. Sleep:
   - Prioritize getting enough quality sleep, as this is when your skin does much of its repair work

Remember, a holistic approach that addresses both internal and external factors is often most effective for managing eczema.

The Importance of Patience and Self-Compassion

Developing an effective skincare routine for eczema is often a process of trial and error. It's important to:

1. Be Patient:
    - It can take time to see results from a new routine or product
    - Don't expect overnight miracles

2. Practice Self-Compassion:
    - Eczema can be frustrating, but remember it's not your fault
    - Treat yourself with kindness and understanding

3. Celebrate Small Victories:
    - Acknowledge improvements, no matter how small
    - Every step towards better skin health is a success

4. Seek Support:
    - Connect with others who have eczema
    - Don't hesitate to reach out to your healthcare provider if you're struggling

Conclusion: Your Skin, Your Routine

Developing an effective skincare routine is a crucial part of managing eczema. By understanding the principles of gentle cleansing, effective moisturizing, proper treatment application, and adequate protection, you can create a routine that works for your unique skin.

Remember these key points:
    - Consistency is crucial in skincare for eczema
    - Choose products carefully, focusing on gentle, fragrance-free options
    - Moisturizing is the cornerstone of eczema skincare
    - Adjust your routine as needed based on your skin's changing needs
    - Be patient and kind to yourself as you navigate your skincare journey

Your skin is unique, and what works best for you may take some time to discover. But with patience, persistence, and the guidance of your healthcare provider, you can develop a skincare routine that helps manage your eczema and promotes overall skin health.

By taking control of your skincare routine, you're not just managing symptoms—you're actively participating in your own healing process. This empowerment, combined with proper medical care, can make a significant difference in living well with eczema.

CHAPTER 10

E czema Through the Life Stages

Eczema is a chronic condition that can affect individuals at any age, from infancy to late adulthood. However, its presentation, triggers, and management can vary significantly across different life stages. In this chapter, we'll explore how eczema manifests and is managed during key periods of life: infancy and childhood, adolescence, adulthood, and in seniors.

Infant and Childhood Eczema

Eczema often first appears in infancy or early childhood, with up to 20% of children affected. This early-onset eczema is typically atopic dermatitis, the most common form of eczema.

Presentation in Infants (0-2 years):
- Often appears around 3-6 months of age
- Commonly affects the face, particularly the cheeks and chin
- May also appear on the scalp, trunk, and extremities
- Skin may appear red, weepy, and crusty

Presentation in Young Children (2-12 years):
- Often affects the creases of elbows and knees
- May also affect the neck, wrists, and ankles

- Skin may become drier, thicker, and more likely to show signs of scratching

Key Considerations for Infant and Childhood Eczema:

1. Diagnosis:
   - A pediatrician or dermatologist can usually diagnose eczema based on the appearance of the skin and family history
   - No specific test is required for diagnosis

2. Triggers:
   - Food allergies are more commonly associated with eczema in young children
   - Common triggers include cow's milk, eggs, peanuts, and soy
   - Environmental factors like dust mites, pet dander, and certain fabrics can also trigger flares

3. Treatment Approach:
   - Gentle skincare is crucial: use mild, fragrance-free products
   - Regular moisturizing is key, especially after bathing
   - Topical corticosteroids may be prescribed for flare-ups, but use should be carefully monitored
   - Topical calcineurin inhibitors might be used, especially for sensitive areas like the face
   - Antihistamines may help with itching and sleep disturbance

4. Special Considerations:
   - Prevent scratching: keep nails short, use mittens for infants if necessary
   - Be cautious with elimination diets: consult a pediatrician or allergist before removing foods from a child's diet
   - Watch for signs of skin infection, which can be more common in children with eczema

5. Education and Support:
   - Educate caregivers and family members about eczema management
   - Teach children age-appropriate ways to care for their skin
   - Consider joining support groups for families dealing with childhood eczema

6. Long-term Outlook:
   - Many children outgrow eczema by adolescence
   - However, some will continue to have symptoms into adulthood
   - Early, consistent treatment may help improve long-term outcomes

Adolescent Eczema

Adolescence brings unique challenges for individuals with eczema, including hormonal changes, increased stress, and the psychological impact of visible skin conditions.

Presentation in Adolescents:
   - May persist from childhood or develop for the first time
   - Often affects similar areas as in childhood (elbow and knee creases)
   - Can also affect the face, neck, and hands
   - May become more severe due to hormonal changes

Key Considerations for Adolescent Eczema:

1. Hormonal Influences:
   - Hormonal changes during puberty can affect eczema
   - Some adolescents may experience worsening symptoms
   - Others might see improvement as they go through puberty

2. Psychological Impact:
   - Visible skin conditions can significantly affect self-esteem and social interactions

- Stress about appearance can, in turn, exacerbate eczema symptoms

3. Treatment Adherence:
  - Adolescents may struggle with consistently following treatment regimens
  - Education about the importance of regular skincare is crucial

4. Lifestyle Factors:
  - Increased participation in sports and physical activities may impact eczema management
  - Sweating can exacerbate symptoms, necessitating proper post-exercise skincare

5. Diet and Nutrition:
  - Dietary changes common in adolescence (e.g., increased consumption of processed foods) may impact eczema
  - Education about skin-healthy eating habits is important

6. Stress Management:
  - Academic and social pressures can increase stress, potentially triggering flares
  - Teaching stress management techniques is crucial

7. Treatment Approach:
  - Similar to childhood, but with increased emphasis on self-management
  - Topical treatments remain the mainstay, but systemic treatments might be considered for severe cases
  - Sun protection becomes increasingly important

8. Transition of Care:
  - Adolescents should be encouraged to take increasing responsibility for their eczema management
  - Gradual transition from pediatric to adult healthcare providers may begin

Adult-Onset Eczema

While many adults with eczema have had the condition since childhood, some experience adult-onset eczema, developing symptoms for the first time in adulthood.

Presentation in Adults:
  - Can affect any part of the body, but commonly involves the hands, eyelids, and flexural areas
    - May be more diffuse and less well-defined than in childhood eczema
    - Skin may be extremely dry, scaly, and prone to cracking

Key Considerations for Adult Eczema:

1. Diagnosis:
  - Adult-onset eczema can be challenging to diagnose as it may resemble other skin conditions
  - A dermatologist may perform patch testing to rule out allergic contact dermatitis

2. Triggers:
  - Occupational exposures become more significant (e.g., frequent hand washing, exposure to chemicals)
    - Stress often plays a major role in adult eczema
    - Environmental factors, including climate and pollution, can impact symptoms

3. Treatment Approach:
  - Similar to other age groups, with an emphasis on topical treatments and skincare
    - Systemic treatments may be considered for severe or resistant cases
    - Phototherapy can be an effective option for some adults

4. Comorbidities:
   - Adults with eczema may have higher rates of other health issues, including cardiovascular disease and depression
   - Comprehensive health management is important

5. Lifestyle Management:
   - Balancing eczema care with work and family responsibilities can be challenging
   - Stress management techniques are crucial

6. Pregnancy Considerations:
   - Eczema can change during pregnancy, improving for some and worsening for others
   - Some treatments may need to be adjusted during pregnancy and breastfeeding

7. Occupational Impact:
   - Eczema, particularly hand eczema, can significantly impact work in certain professions
   - Occupational counseling and workplace accommodations may be necessary

8. Psychological Support:
   - The chronic nature of eczema can take a toll on mental health
   - Access to psychological support should be part of comprehensive care

Eczema in Seniors

While eczema often improves with age, some individuals continue to experience symptoms into their senior years, and some may develop eczema for the first time in late adulthood.

Presentation in Seniors:

- May be a continuation of long-standing eczema or new-onset
- Often affects the face, neck, and hands
- Skin may be extremely dry and prone to cracking
- Itching can be severe and significantly impact quality of life

Key Considerations for Eczema in Seniors:

1. Skin Changes:
  - Age-related skin changes, including decreased oil production and thinning skin, can exacerbate eczema
  - Skin becomes more fragile and prone to injury

2. Diagnosis:
  - Differential diagnosis is important, as other skin conditions become more common with age
  - Skin biopsies may be necessary to rule out other conditions like cutaneous T-cell lymphoma

3. Comorbidities:
  - Other health conditions common in seniors can complicate eczema management
  - Medications for other conditions may impact eczema or interact with eczema treatments

4. Treatment Approach:
  - Gentle skincare becomes even more critical
  - Topical treatments remain first-line, but care must be taken due to increased skin fragility
  - Systemic treatments must be used cautiously due to potential side effects and drug interactions

5. Lifestyle Factors:
  - Reduced mobility may impact skincare routines

- Changes in living situations (e.g., moving to assisted living) may introduce new triggers

6. Nutritional Considerations:
   - Ensuring adequate nutrition is crucial for skin health
   - Vitamin D supplementation may be beneficial, especially for seniors with limited sun exposure

7. Prevention of Complications:
   - Seniors with eczema are at increased risk of skin infections
   - Regular skin checks and prompt treatment of any breaks in the skin are important

8. Quality of Life:
   - Chronic itching can significantly impact sleep and overall quality of life
   - Comprehensive management should address both physical symptoms and quality of life concerns

Special Considerations Across Life Stages

While eczema management has unique aspects at each life stage, some considerations span across all ages:

1. Individualized Care:
   - Eczema presentation and triggers can vary greatly between individuals
   - Treatment plans should be tailored to each person's specific needs and circumstances

2. Comprehensive Approach:
   - Eczema management should address not just skin symptoms, but overall health and well-being
   - A multidisciplinary approach involving dermatologists, allergists, primary care providers, and mental health professionals may be beneficial

3. Education and Self-Management:
   - At all ages, education about eczema and its management is crucial
   - Encouraging age-appropriate self-management skills can improve outcomes

4. Ongoing Monitoring:
   - Regular follow-up is important to assess treatment effectiveness and adjust as needed
   - Monitoring for potential treatment side effects is crucial, especially with long-term use of certain medications

5. Psychosocial Support:
   - The impact of eczema on quality of life should be addressed at all ages
   - Access to support groups and mental health resources can be beneficial

6. Addressing Comorbidities:
   - Be aware of conditions commonly associated with eczema, such as asthma, allergies, and depression
   - Comprehensive care should address these associated conditions

7. Environmental Modifications:
   - Identifying and managing environmental triggers is important at all life stages
   - This may involve changes to home environment, clothing choices, and daily routines

8. Nutrition and Diet:
   - While dietary triggers can change over time, maintaining a balanced, nutrient-rich diet is important for skin health at all ages

9. Stress Management:
   - Stress can exacerbate eczema at any age
   - Age-appropriate stress management techniques should be part of eczema

care

10. Sleep Quality:
   - Eczema can significantly impact sleep, which in turn affects overall health and eczema symptoms
   - Addressing sleep issues should be a priority at all life stages

Transitions of Care

As individuals with eczema move through different life stages, transitions in care are important to manage:

1. Pediatric to Adult Care:
   - Transition should be gradual, starting in early adolescence
   - Focus on building self-management skills and understanding of the condition
   - Ensure continuity of care during the transition

2. Reproductive Years:
   - Women with eczema should discuss family planning with their healthcare providers
   - Some eczema treatments may need to be adjusted before, during, and after pregnancy

3. Entering Senior Years:
   - As individuals age, their eczema care may need to be coordinated with management of other health conditions
   - Consider the impact of age-related changes on eczema management

Emerging Treatments and Research

Research into eczema treatment continues to evolve, with new therapies emerging that may benefit individuals at various life stages:

1. Biologics:
 - Targeted therapies like dupilumab have shown promise for moderate to severe atopic dermatitis in adults and adolescents
 - Research is ongoing for use in younger children

2. JAK Inhibitors:
 - Both oral and topical JAK inhibitors are being studied for eczema treatment
 - These may offer new options for individuals with treatment-resistant eczema

3. Microbiome-Based Therapies:
 - Research into the skin microbiome may lead to new treatments that restore balance to the skin's microbial ecosystem

4. Gene Therapy:
 - As we understand more about the genetic basis of eczema, gene-targeted therapies may become possible in the future

5. Personalized Medicine:
 - Advances in understanding different eczema subtypes may lead to more personalized treatment approaches

As new treatments become available, it will be important to understand their safety and efficacy across different age groups.

Conclusion: A Lifelong Approach to Eczema Management

Eczema is a chronic condition that can affect individuals throughout their lives, presenting unique challenges at each life stage. From the delicate skin of infancy to the complex health considerations of senior years, managing eczema requires an approach that adapts to changing needs and circumstances.

Key takeaways:

- Eczema presentation and triggers can change significantly across life stages

- Treatment approaches must be tailored not just to the individual, but to their current life stage

- Comprehensive care should address not just skin symptoms, but overall health and quality of life

- Transitions between life stages require careful management to ensure continuity of care

- Emerging treatments offer hope for improved management across all age groups

By understanding how eczema manifests and is managed at different life stages, individuals with eczema and their healthcare providers can work together to develop effective, age-appropriate management strategies. This lifelong approach to eczema care can help individuals not just manage their symptoms, but thrive at every stage of life.

Remember, while eczema is a chronic condition, it doesn't define a person. With proper care, support, and a positive outlook, individuals with eczema can lead full, active lives at any age. The key is to stay informed, work closely with healthcare providers, and remain adaptable as needs change throughout life's journey.

CHAPTER 11

Living with Eczema: Psychological and Social Aspects

While much of our focus has been on the physical symptoms and management of eczema, it's crucial to address the significant psychological and social impact this chronic condition can have. In this chapter, we'll explore the emotional challenges of living with eczema, discuss coping strategies, and provide guidance on navigating social situations and relationships.

The Emotional Toll of Eczema

Living with eczema can be emotionally challenging. The unpredictable nature of flare-ups, the constant need for management, and the visible nature of the condition can all take a toll on mental health.

Common emotional challenges include:

1. Anxiety:
   - Worry about potential flare-ups
   - Anxiety in social situations due to visible symptoms
   - Concern about long-term health implications

2. Depression:
   - Feelings of hopelessness about managing the condition

- Low mood related to chronic discomfort and sleep disturbance
- Social isolation due to embarrassment about skin appearance

3. Frustration and Anger:
    - Irritation with constant itching and discomfort
    - Frustration with treatment regimens and perceived lack of progress
    - Anger at the unfairness of having a chronic condition

4. Low Self-Esteem:
    - Negative body image due to visible skin symptoms
    - Feeling self-conscious in social or intimate situations
    - Reduced confidence in personal and professional life

5. Stress:
    - The demands of managing eczema can be stressful in themselves
    - Stress can, in turn, exacerbate eczema symptoms, creating a vicious cycle

6. Sleep Disturbance:
    - Itching and discomfort can significantly impact sleep quality
    - Poor sleep can affect mood, cognitive function, and overall quality of life

7. Guilt:
    - Parents of children with eczema may feel guilty, especially if there's a family history
    - Individuals may feel guilty about the impact of their condition on family members

Recognizing these emotional challenges is the first step in addressing them. It's important to understand that these feelings are normal and valid responses to living with a chronic condition.

Coping Strategies

Developing effective coping strategies is crucial for managing the psychological impact of eczema. Here are some approaches that can help:

1. Education and Understanding:
   - Learn as much as you can about eczema
   - Understanding your condition can help reduce anxiety and increase a sense of control

2. Mindfulness and Relaxation Techniques:
   - Practice mindfulness meditation to reduce stress and improve emotional regulation
   - Try relaxation techniques like deep breathing or progressive muscle relaxation

3. Cognitive Behavioral Therapy (CBT):
   - CBT can help change negative thought patterns and behaviors
   - It can be particularly helpful for managing stress, anxiety, and depression related to eczema

4. Stress Management:
   - Identify personal stress triggers and develop strategies to manage them
   - Regular exercise, adequate sleep, and healthy eating can all contribute to stress reduction

5. Support Groups:
   - Connecting with others who have eczema can provide emotional support and practical advice
   - Online forums and local support groups can be valuable resources

6. Journaling:
   - Keeping a journal can help process emotions and identify patterns in symptoms and triggers
   - It can also be a useful tool for tracking treatment effectiveness

7. Creative Expression:
   - Art, music, writing, or other creative activities can be therapeutic outlets for emotions

8. Professional Help:
   - Don't hesitate to seek help from a mental health professional if you're struggling
   - Some therapists specialize in working with individuals with chronic health conditions

9. Positive Self-Talk:
   - Practice reframing negative thoughts into more positive, realistic ones
   - Remind yourself of your strengths and accomplishments beyond your skin condition

10. Self-Care Activities:
    - Engage in activities that bring you joy and relaxation
    - Make time for hobbies and interests unrelated to eczema

Remember, coping with eczema is an ongoing process. It's okay to have bad days, and it's important to be kind to yourself as you navigate the challenges of living with a chronic condition.

Building Self-Esteem

Eczema can significantly impact self-esteem, particularly when symptoms are visible. Here are strategies for building and maintaining a positive self-image:

1. Focus on Your Whole Self:
   - Remember that you are much more than your skin condition
   - Make a list of your positive qualities, skills, and accomplishments

2. Challenge Beauty Standards:
   - Question societal beauty norms that prioritize "perfect" skin
   - Seek out and celebrate diverse representations of beauty

3. Practice Self-Compassion:
   - Treat yourself with the same kindness you would offer a friend
   - Acknowledge that living with eczema is challenging, and you're doing your best

4. Positive Affirmations:
   - Use positive self-talk to counteract negative thoughts about your appearance
   - Create and repeat affirmations that resonate with you

5. Embrace Your Uniqueness:
   - View your eczema as part of what makes you unique, not a flaw
   - Consider sharing your story to empower others and build confidence

6. Focus on What Your Body Can Do:
   - Appreciate your body for its functions and abilities, not just its appearance
   - Engage in physical activities that make you feel strong and capable

7. Surround Yourself with Support:
   - Spend time with people who appreciate you for who you are
   - Distance yourself from individuals who make negative comments about your appearance

8. Seek Professional Help:
   - A therapist can provide strategies for improving self-esteem and body image

Building self-esteem is an ongoing process. Be patient with yourself and celebrate small victories along the way.

Navigating Social Situations

Eczema can present challenges in social situations, but with the right strategies, you can maintain an active social life:

1. Educate Others:
   - Be prepared to explain eczema to others in simple terms
   - Helping people understand your condition can reduce misconceptions and increase support

2. Plan Ahead:
   - Bring necessary items (like moisturizer) when going out
   - Choose clothing that's comfortable and doesn't irritate your skin

3. Choose Activities Wisely:
   - Opt for activities that won't exacerbate your symptoms
   - Be open with friends about your needs and limitations

4. Develop a "Flare-Up Plan":
   - Have strategies ready for managing unexpected flare-ups in social situations
   - This might include having a change of clothes or knowing where to find a quiet spot to apply medication

5. Practice Assertiveness:
   - Learn to communicate your needs clearly and respectfully
   - It's okay to say no to activities that might trigger your eczema

6. Find Supportive Communities:
   - Seek out groups or events where you feel comfortable and understood
   - This might include support groups or activities for individuals with chronic health conditions

7. Address Misconceptions:
   - Be prepared to correct common misconceptions about eczema (e.g., that it's contagious)
   - Use these moments as opportunities for education

8. Focus on Connections:
   - Remember that true friends will value you regardless of your skin's appearance
   - Concentrate on building meaningful relationships based on shared interests and values

Relationships and Intimacy

Eczema can impact personal relationships, including romantic partnerships. Here are some strategies for navigating relationships and intimacy:

1. Open Communication:
   - Be honest with partners about your condition and its impact
   - Discuss how eczema affects you physically and emotionally

2. Educate Your Partner:
   - Help your partner understand eczema, its triggers, and its management
   - Involve them in your care routine if you're comfortable doing so

3. Addressing Intimacy Concerns:
   - Discuss any concerns about physical intimacy openly
   - Work together to find ways to be intimate that are comfortable for you

4. Managing Flare-Ups:
   - Have a plan for managing flare-ups that might impact your relationship
   - This might include having separate bedding or adjusting shared activities

5. Emotional Support:

- Express your emotional needs to your partner
- Be open about when you need extra support or understanding

6. Maintaining Independence:
   - While support is important, maintain some independence in managing your condition
   - This can prevent feelings of over-reliance or resentment

7. Couples Counseling:
   - Consider couples therapy if eczema is causing significant strain on your relationship
   - A therapist can help you communicate effectively and develop coping strategies as a couple

Remember, a supportive partner can be a tremendous asset in managing eczema. Open, honest communication is key to maintaining a healthy relationship while living with a chronic condition.

Workplace Considerations

Managing eczema in the workplace presents unique challenges. Here are some strategies:

1. Know Your Rights:
   - Familiarize yourself with disability laws in your country
   - Understand what reasonable accommodations you might be entitled to

2. Communicate with Employers:
   - Be upfront about your condition and any needs you might have
   - Discuss potential accommodations that could help you perform your job effectively

3. Manage Stress:

- Workplace stress can exacerbate eczema symptoms
- Develop stress management techniques specific to your work environment

4. Create a Skin-Friendly Workspace:
   - Use a humidifier if dry air is a problem
   - Ensure your work area is clean and free of potential irritants

5. Plan for Flare-Ups:
   - Have a plan for managing unexpected flare-ups at work
   - This might include keeping medication or moisturizer at your desk

6. Educate Coworkers:
   - Consider sharing information about your condition with colleagues to increase understanding
   - Address any misconceptions about eczema

7. Choose Appropriate Work Attire:
   - Opt for comfortable, breathable clothing that doesn't irritate your skin
   - If you have a uniform, discuss possible modifications if needed

8. Consider Your Career Path:
   - If your current job exacerbates your eczema, consider roles or industries that might be more suitable
   - Consult with a career counselor if you're considering a change

Remember, you have the right to a work environment that doesn't exacerbate your health condition. Don't hesitate to advocate for your needs.

Parenting with Eczema

For parents with eczema, managing their condition while caring for children can be challenging. Here are some strategies:

1. Educate Your Children:

  - Explain your condition to your children in age-appropriate terms

  - Help them understand why you might need to do things differently sometimes

2. Manage Expectations:

  - Be realistic about what you can do, especially during flare-ups

  - It's okay to adjust family activities based on your needs

3. Seek Support:

  - Don't hesitate to ask for help from partners, family members, or friends when needed

  - Consider joining support groups for parents with chronic health conditions

4. Model Self-Care:

  - Show your children the importance of taking care of your health

  - This can be a valuable lesson in self-care and resilience

5. Adapt Activities:

  - Find ways to engage with your children that don't exacerbate your symptoms

  - Be creative in finding new ways to play and bond

6. Address Emotional Impacts:

  - Be open about your feelings with age-appropriate honesty

  - Ensure children don't feel responsible for your condition or its management

7. Prepare for Emergencies:

  - Have a plan for severe flare-ups, including childcare arrangements if needed

Remember, taking care of yourself is an important part of being a good parent. It's not selfish to prioritize your health needs.

Eczema and Mental Health: When to Seek Help

While it's normal to experience emotional challenges when living with eczema, sometimes professional help is needed. Consider seeking help from a mental health professional if:

1. You're experiencing persistent feelings of sadness, hopelessness, or anxiety
2. Eczema is significantly impacting your daily functioning or quality of life
3. You're having thoughts of self-harm or suicide
4. You're struggling to adhere to your treatment plan due to emotional factors
5. You're using unhealthy coping mechanisms (e.g., substance abuse)
6. Your relationships are suffering due to eczema-related stress
7. You're experiencing significant sleep disturbances
8. You're having difficulty accepting your condition

Remember, seeking help is a sign of strength, not weakness. Mental health professionals can provide valuable tools and support for managing the psychological aspects of living with a chronic condition.

Building Resilience

Resilience – the ability to adapt and bounce back from adversity – is crucial for living well with eczema. Here are some ways to build resilience:

1. Develop a Growth Mindset:

- View challenges as opportunities for learning and growth
- Embrace the idea that you can develop new coping skills over time

2. Build a Strong Support Network:
    - Cultivate relationships with understanding friends and family
    - Connect with others who have eczema for shared support

3. Practice Self-Compassion:
    - Be kind to yourself, especially during flare-ups
    - Recognize that everyone faces challenges, and it's okay to struggle
sometimes

4. Set Realistic Goals:
    - Break larger goals into smaller, manageable steps
    - Celebrate small victories in managing your condition

5. Maintain Perspective:
    - Remember that flare-ups are temporary
    - Focus on aspects of your life beyond your skin condition

6. Develop Problem-Solving Skills:
    - Approach challenges with a solution-focused mindset
    - Be willing to try different strategies to find what works best for you

7. Practice Gratitude:
    - Regularly acknowledge things you're grateful for, even during difficult
times
    - This can help maintain a positive outlook

8. Engage in Meaningful Activities:
    - Pursue hobbies and interests that bring you joy and fulfillment
    - Volunteering or helping others can also boost resilience

Building resilience is an ongoing process. Be patient with yourself and recognize that developing these skills takes time.

Conclusion: Thriving, Not Just Surviving

Living with eczema presents numerous psychological and social challenges, but it's possible to not just manage these challenges, but to thrive in spite of them. By developing effective coping strategies, building self-esteem, navigating social situations skillfully, and fostering resilience, individuals with eczema can lead full, satisfying lives.

Key takeaways:
- Acknowledge the emotional impact of eczema
- Develop a toolkit of coping strategies that work for you
- Build self-esteem that goes beyond skin appearance
- Communicate openly about your needs in relationships and work settings
- Seek professional help when needed
- Focus on building resilience to face challenges effectively

Remember, your worth is not determined by the condition of your skin. Eczema may be a part of your life, but it doesn't define you. With the right support, strategies, and mindset, you can live a rich, fulfilling life while managing your eczema effectively.

By addressing both the physical and psychological aspects of eczema, you're taking a holistic approach to your health and well-being. This comprehensive care can lead to better outcomes, improved quality of life, and a sense of empowerment in managing your condition.

Living well with eczema is a journey, not a destination. Be patient with yourself, celebrate your progress, and remember that you have the strength and resilience to face whatever challenges come your way.

CHAPTER 12

Eczema and Comorbid Conditions

While eczema, particularly atopic dermatitis, is often viewed primarily as a skin condition, it's increasingly recognized as a systemic disorder that can be associated with various other health issues. In this chapter, we'll explore the common comorbidities associated with eczema, discuss the potential underlying connections, and consider how these associations impact overall health management for individuals with eczema.

The Atopic March

One of the most well-established associations with eczema is the concept of the "atopic march." This term describes the typical progression of atopic diseases:

1. Eczema (usually the first to appear, often in infancy)
2. Food allergies
3. Asthma
4. Allergic rhinitis (hay fever)

While not every individual with eczema will experience all of these conditions, there's a significant overlap. Understanding this progression can help in early intervention and management of these related conditions.

Key points about the atopic march:
  - It highlights the systemic nature of atopic diseases
  - Early-onset, severe eczema is associated with a higher risk of developing other atopic conditions
  - Management of one condition may impact the others
  - A coordinated approach involving different specialists (dermatologists, allergists, pulmonologists) may be beneficial

Asthma and Allergic Rhinitis

The link between eczema, asthma, and allergic rhinitis is well-established:

1. Asthma:
  - Up to 80% of children with atopic dermatitis develop asthma later in life
  - Shared genetic factors and immune system dysfunction contribute to this association
  - Both conditions involve inflammation and hypersensitivity reactions

Management considerations:
  - Regular lung function monitoring for eczema patients
  - Considering the impact of asthma medications on skin health
  - Addressing environmental triggers that may affect both conditions

2. Allergic Rhinitis:
  - Also known as hay fever, it frequently co-occurs with eczema
  - Shared triggers (like dust mites or pollen) can exacerbate both conditions

Management considerations:
  - Allergen avoidance strategies can benefit both conditions
  - Antihistamines used for allergic rhinitis may also help with eczema-

related itching
   - Considering the impact of nasal corticosteroids on overall steroid load

Food Allergies and Eczema

The relationship between food allergies and eczema is complex and often misunderstood:

Key points:
   - Food allergies are more common in children with eczema
   - Not all food sensitivities in eczema patients are true allergies
   - The relationship can be bidirectional: eczema can increase the risk of developing food allergies, and food allergies can exacerbate eczema symptoms

Common food allergens associated with eczema:
   - Cow's milk
   - Eggs
   - Peanuts
   - Tree nuts
   - Soy
   - Wheat
   - Fish and shellfish

Management considerations:
   - Proper allergy testing is crucial before eliminating foods from the diet
   - Work with an allergist or dietitian to ensure nutritional needs are met if foods are eliminated
   - Consider the timing of food introduction in infants with eczema
   - Be aware that food allergies can develop or resolve over time

Mental Health Conditions

The psychological impact of eczema can be significant, and there's a higher prevalence of certain mental health conditions among individuals with eczema:

1. Depression:
   - Individuals with eczema have a higher risk of developing depression
   - Chronic itch, sleep disturbance, and the visible nature of the condition contribute to this risk

2. Anxiety:
   - Anxiety disorders are more common in people with eczema
   - The unpredictable nature of flare-ups can contribute to anxiety

3. Attention Deficit Hyperactivity Disorder (ADHD):
   - Some studies have found a higher prevalence of ADHD in children with eczema
   - The link may be related to sleep disturbance or shared inflammatory processes

Management considerations:
   - Regular screening for mental health issues
   - Incorporating stress management techniques into eczema care
   - Considering the psychological impact when choosing treatments
   - Referral to mental health professionals when needed

Cardiovascular Health and Eczema

Emerging research suggests a potential link between eczema and cardiovascular health:

Key points:
   - Some studies have found an increased risk of cardiovascular disease in adults with eczema

- The link may be related to chronic inflammation or shared risk factors
- Sleep disturbance and reduced physical activity due to eczema may also play a role

Management considerations:
- Regular cardiovascular risk assessment for adults with eczema
- Promoting heart-healthy lifestyle choices as part of overall eczema management
- Considering the cardiovascular impact of certain eczema treatments (e.g., long-term oral corticosteroid use)

Autoimmune Disorders

There's growing evidence of an association between eczema and certain autoimmune disorders:

1. Alopecia Areata:
   - An autoimmune condition causing hair loss
   - More common in individuals with eczema

2. Vitiligo:
   - An autoimmune condition causing loss of skin pigmentation
   - Has been found to occur more frequently in people with eczema

3. Inflammatory Bowel Disease (IBD):
   - Some studies suggest a higher prevalence of IBD in individuals with eczema
   - The link may be related to shared immune system dysfunction

Management considerations:
- Be aware of symptoms of these conditions for early detection
- Consider the impact of treatments for one condition on the others
- A multidisciplinary approach may be beneficial for managing multiple

autoimmune conditions

Skin Infections

People with eczema are more susceptible to certain skin infections due to the compromised skin barrier and immune system alterations:

1. Staphylococcus aureus:
   - Up to 90% of eczema patients have S. aureus colonization on their skin
   - Can exacerbate eczema symptoms and trigger flares

2. Herpes Simplex Virus (HSV):
   - Can cause eczema herpeticum, a serious condition requiring prompt treatment
   - More common in individuals with poorly controlled eczema

3. Molluscum Contagiosum:
   - A viral skin infection more common in children with eczema
   - Can be more widespread and persistent in eczema patients

Management considerations:
   - Regular skin checks for signs of infection
   - Proper skincare to maintain skin barrier function
   - Prompt treatment of infections when they occur
   - Consider antimicrobial treatments in severe or recurrent cases

Sleep Disorders

Sleep disturbance is a common issue for people with eczema, but it can also lead to more severe sleep disorders:

1. Insomnia:
   - Difficulty falling asleep or staying asleep is common in eczema patients

- Can be due to itching, discomfort, or anxiety

2. Sleep Apnea:
   - Some studies suggest a higher prevalence of sleep apnea in individuals with eczema
   - The link may be related to shared inflammatory processes or the impact of eczema treatments

Management considerations:
   - Addressing itch and discomfort to improve sleep quality
   - Implementing good sleep hygiene practices
   - Considering sleep studies if sleep apnea is suspected
   - Recognizing the bidirectional relationship: poor sleep can worsen eczema, and eczema can disrupt sleep

Gastrointestinal Issues

There's growing interest in the gut-skin axis and how gastrointestinal health may relate to eczema:

1. Irritable Bowel Syndrome (IBS):
   - Some studies suggest a higher prevalence of IBS in individuals with eczema
   - The link may be related to shared immune system dysfunction or the gut microbiome

2. Celiac Disease:
   - There may be a slightly increased risk of celiac disease in people with eczema
   - Gluten sensitivity (even without celiac disease) may exacerbate eczema symptoms in some individuals

3. Eosinophilic Esophagitis:

- A chronic allergic condition of the esophagus
- More common in individuals with eczema and other atopic conditions

Management considerations:
- Be aware of gastrointestinal symptoms and seek appropriate evaluation
- Consider the role of diet in managing both eczema and gastrointestinal issues
- Explore the potential benefits of probiotics for both skin and gut health

Obesity and Metabolic Syndrome

There's evidence of a bidirectional relationship between eczema and obesity:

Key points:
- Obesity may increase the risk of developing eczema
- Eczema may increase the risk of obesity, possibly due to reduced physical activity or the effects of certain treatments
- Metabolic syndrome (a cluster of conditions including high blood pressure, high blood sugar, abnormal cholesterol levels, and excess abdominal fat) may be more common in adults with eczema

Management considerations:
- Promoting a healthy diet and regular physical activity as part of eczema management
- Considering the impact of weight on eczema symptoms and treatment effectiveness
- Monitoring for components of metabolic syndrome in adults with eczema

Bone Health

Long-term use of certain eczema treatments, particularly oral corticosteroids, can impact bone health:

Key points:
  - Prolonged corticosteroid use can lead to decreased bone density
  - Children with severe eczema may have slower growth and delayed puberty, which can affect bone development

Management considerations:
  - Monitoring bone density in individuals on long-term corticosteroid treatment
  - Ensuring adequate calcium and vitamin D intake
  - Promoting weight-bearing exercise for bone health
  - Considering alternative treatments to minimize long-term corticosteroid use

Eye Conditions

Several eye conditions are more common in individuals with eczema:

1. Atopic Keratoconjunctivitis:
  - Chronic inflammation of the conjunctiva and cornea
  - Can lead to vision impairment if not properly managed

2. Keratoconus:
  - A condition where the cornea thins and bulges outward
  - More common in individuals with atopic conditions, including eczema

3. Cataracts:
  - Long-term use of oral corticosteroids can increase the risk of cataracts
  - Some studies suggest an increased risk of cataracts in eczema patients even without corticosteroid use

Management considerations:
  - Regular eye exams for individuals with eczema
  - Proper care when applying eczema treatments near the eyes

- Considering the ocular impact of long-term corticosteroid use

Managing Multiple Conditions: An Integrated Approach

Given the range of potential comorbidities, managing eczema often requires an integrated, multidisciplinary approach:

1. Comprehensive Assessment:
   - Regular screening for common comorbidities
   - Considering the whole person, not just the skin symptoms

2. Coordinated Care:
   - Collaboration between different specialists (dermatologists, allergists, pulmonologists, gastroenterologists, mental health professionals)
   - Ensuring treatments for different conditions are complementary, not conflicting

3. Patient Education:
   - Helping individuals understand the interconnected nature of their health issues
   - Empowering patients to recognize symptoms of potential comorbidities

4. Lifestyle Management:
   - Promoting overall health through diet, exercise, stress management, and sleep hygiene
   - Addressing modifiable risk factors for comorbid conditions

5. Personalized Treatment Plans:
   - Tailoring treatments to address multiple conditions simultaneously when possible
   - Considering the impact of treatments for one condition on others

6. Regular Monitoring:

- Ongoing assessment of both eczema and comorbid conditions
- Adjusting management strategies as needed based on overall health status

7. Holistic Approach to Triggers:
 - Identifying and managing triggers that may affect multiple conditions (e.g., stress, certain foods, environmental factors)

8. Supporting Mental Health:
 - Recognizing the psychological impact of managing multiple health conditions
 - Providing resources for mental health support

9. Considering Long-Term Health Impacts:
 - Making treatment decisions with an awareness of potential long-term health effects
 - Balancing the management of acute symptoms with long-term health considerations

The Role of the Patient in Managing Comorbidities

Individuals with eczema play a crucial role in managing their overall health:

1. Self-Awareness:
 - Learn to recognize symptoms of potential comorbidities
 - Keep track of any new or changing symptoms

2. Open Communication:
 - Share all health concerns with healthcare providers, even if they seem unrelated to eczema
 - Provide a complete health history to all specialists involved in care

3. Adherence to Treatment Plans:
 - Follow treatment plans for all conditions

- Communicate any difficulties in managing multiple treatments

4. Lifestyle Management:
   - Take an active role in implementing healthy lifestyle changes
   - Recognize the impact of lifestyle factors on overall health

5. Self-Advocacy:
   - Ask questions about potential comorbidities and screening recommendations
   - Seek referrals to specialists when needed

6. Emotional Self-Care:
   - Acknowledge the emotional impact of managing multiple health conditions
   - Seek support when feeling overwhelmed

Conclusion: A Holistic View of Eczema and Health

Understanding the relationship between eczema and various comorbid conditions is crucial for comprehensive health management. While the presence of these associations can seem daunting, awareness allows for early detection, proactive management, and better overall health outcomes.

Key takeaways:
   - Eczema is often part of a broader picture of atopic and immune-mediated conditions
   - Regular screening and awareness of potential comorbidities is important
   - An integrated, multidisciplinary approach to healthcare is often beneficial
   - Lifestyle factors play a crucial role in managing both eczema and associated conditions
   - Patients play an active role in managing their overall health

By taking a holistic view of health, individuals with eczema can work with their healthcare providers to develop comprehensive management strategies that address not just their skin symptoms, but their overall well-being. This approach can lead to improved quality of life, better health outcomes, and a sense of empowerment in managing complex health needs.

Remember, while eczema and its associated conditions present challenges, many individuals successfully manage multiple health issues and lead full, active lives. With the right care, support, and self-management strategies, it's possible to thrive while navigating the complexities of eczema and its comorbidities.

CHAPTER 13

Emerging Treatments and Research

The field of eczema treatment is rapidly evolving, with new therapies and approaches constantly being developed and tested. In this chapter, we'll explore the cutting-edge research and emerging treatments that are shaping the future of eczema care. From targeted biologics to microbiome-based therapies, we'll discuss the most promising developments and what they might mean for individuals living with eczema.

Biologics: The New Frontier

Biologic drugs represent one of the most significant advancements in eczema treatment in recent years. These therapies target specific components of the immune system involved in the inflammatory process of eczema.

1. Dupilumab:
   - The first biologic approved for moderate-to-severe atopic dermatitis
   - Targets interleukin-4 (IL-4) and interleukin-13 (IL-13) signaling
   - Has shown significant efficacy in reducing eczema symptoms and improving quality of life

2. Tralokinumab:
   - Specifically targets IL-13
   - Recently approved for moderate-to-severe atopic dermatitis in adults

- Shows promising results in reducing eczema severity and itch

3. Lebrikizumab:
   - Another IL-13 inhibitor in late-stage clinical trials
   - Shows potential for improving skin clearance and reducing itch

4. Nemolizumab:
   - Targets the interleukin-31 (IL-31) receptor, which is heavily involved in itch signaling
   - Shows promise in reducing itch and improving sleep in eczema patients

5. Etokimab:
   - An anti-IL-33 antibody in clinical trials
   - Early results suggest potential in reducing eczema symptoms

Advantages of biologics:
   - Highly targeted approach, potentially reducing side effects
   - Can be effective in cases resistant to traditional therapies
   - May have positive effects on comorbid conditions (e.g., asthma, allergic rhinitis)

Challenges:
   - High cost, which may limit accessibility
   - Long-term safety data still being gathered
   - Require injections, which may be a barrier for some patients

As research continues, we may see more biologics targeting different aspects of the immune response in eczema, potentially offering more personalized treatment options.

JAK Inhibitors: A New Class of Oral Medications

Janus Kinase (JAK) inhibitors represent a new class of oral medications showing promise in eczema treatment:

1. Upadacitinib:
   - Recently approved for moderate-to-severe atopic dermatitis in adults and adolescents
   - Oral medication taken once daily
   - Shows rapid and significant improvement in eczema symptoms

2. Abrocitinib:
   - Another oral JAK inhibitor approved for moderate-to-severe atopic dermatitis
   - Demonstrates fast onset of action in reducing itch and improving skin clearance

3. Baricitinib:
   - Approved in some countries for atopic dermatitis
   - Shows efficacy in improving eczema symptoms and quality of life

Advantages of JAK inhibitors:
   - Oral administration, which may be preferred by some patients
   - Rapid onset of action
   - May address both skin symptoms and itch effectively

Considerations:
   - Potential for more systemic side effects compared to targeted biologics
   - Long-term safety profile still being evaluated
   - Require regular monitoring for potential side effects

Topical JAK inhibitors are also in development, which may offer a more targeted approach with potentially fewer systemic effects.

Microbiome-Based Therapies

Growing understanding of the skin microbiome's role in eczema has led to research into microbiome-based treatments:

1. Topical Microbiome Transplantation:
   - Involves applying beneficial bacteria to the skin
   - Aims to restore a healthy balance of skin microorganisms
   - Early studies show promise in reducing eczema severity

2. Prebiotics and Probiotics:
   - Topical and oral formulations being studied
   - May help promote a healthy skin microbiome
   - Some studies suggest potential in preventing and managing eczema flares

3. Antimicrobial Peptides:
   - Naturally occurring or synthetic peptides that can kill harmful bacteria
   - May help control Staphylococcus aureus overgrowth common in eczema

4. Bacteriophage Therapy:
   - Uses viruses that specifically target harmful bacteria
   - Could potentially offer a more targeted approach than traditional antibiotics

Potential advantages:
   - May offer a more natural approach to managing skin health
   - Could potentially reduce the need for antibiotics
   - Addresses the underlying microbial imbalance in eczema

Challenges:
   - Determining the most effective strains and formulations
   - Ensuring consistent and stable products
   - Long-term effects on skin microbiome still being studied

Barrier Repair Therapies

Enhancing the skin's barrier function is a key focus of eczema research:

1. Advanced Emollients:
   - Formulations that mimic the skin's natural lipid composition
   - May help restore and maintain skin barrier function more effectively than traditional moisturizers

2. Filaggrin Replacement Therapy:
   - Aims to address filaggrin deficiency common in many eczema patients
   - Could potentially correct the underlying barrier dysfunction in eczema

3. Nanotechnology-Based Treatments:
   - Using nanoparticles to deliver moisturizing and anti-inflammatory agents more effectively
   - May improve penetration and efficacy of topical treatments

4. Biomimetic Materials:
   - Synthetic materials designed to mimic the structure and function of healthy skin
   - Could potentially provide temporary barrier protection while the skin heals

These approaches aim to address the fundamental barrier dysfunction in eczema, potentially offering more long-lasting relief and prevention of flares.

Immunomodulators and Small Molecule Inhibitors

Beyond JAK inhibitors, other small molecule drugs are being investigated:

1. PDE4 Inhibitors:
   - Crisaborole is already approved as a topical treatment
   - New formulations and oral PDE4 inhibitors are in development

2. Aryl Hydrocarbon Receptor (AhR) Modulators:
   - Show potential in regulating skin inflammation and barrier function
   - Both topical and oral formulations being studied

3. TSLP Inhibitors:
   - Target thymic stromal lymphopoietin, a key player in the eczema inflammatory cascade
   - Both monoclonal antibodies and small molecule inhibitors in development

4. H4 Receptor Antagonists:
   - Target histamine receptors involved in itch signaling
   - Show promise in reducing itch in eczema patients

These targeted therapies aim to modulate specific aspects of the immune response involved in eczema, potentially offering more precise treatment options.

Gene Therapy and Personalized Medicine

Advancements in genetic research are opening new avenues for eczema treatment:

1. Gene Therapy:
   - Aims to correct genetic mutations associated with eczema (e.g., filaggrin gene mutations)
   - Still in early stages of research, but holds potential for addressing the root cause of eczema in some patients

2. Pharmacogenomics:
   - Studying how genetic variations affect response to eczema treatments
   - Could lead to more personalized treatment selections based on an individual's genetic profile

3. Epigenetic Therapies:
   - Targeting epigenetic modifications that influence eczema development
   - May offer ways to modify gene expression without altering DNA sequence

4. RNA-Based Therapies:
   - Using RNA interference or antisense oligonucleotides to modulate gene expression
   - Could potentially target specific inflammatory pathways in eczema

These approaches hold promise for more personalized and targeted treatments, potentially improving efficacy and reducing side effects.

Novel Drug Delivery Systems

Improving how drugs are delivered to the skin is another area of active research:

1. Microneedle Patches:
   - Painless patches that deliver medication directly into the skin
   - Could improve efficacy and reduce systemic exposure of topical treatments

2. Nanocarriers:
   - Microscopic particles that can carry drugs more effectively into the skin
   - May improve penetration and efficacy of topical treatments

3. Controlled Release Systems:
   - Formulations that release medication slowly over time
   - Could potentially provide more consistent treatment with less frequent application

4. Iontophoresis and Sonophoresis:

- Using electrical current or ultrasound to enhance drug penetration through the skin
- May improve delivery of topical medications, especially in areas with thickened skin

These novel delivery systems aim to enhance the effectiveness of existing and new eczema treatments while potentially reducing side effects and improving ease of use.

Complementary and Alternative Medicine Research

While conventional medical research continues, there's also growing interest in studying complementary and alternative approaches:

1. Chinese Herbal Medicine:
   - Some formulations show promise in clinical trials
   - Research focusing on standardization and understanding mechanisms of action

2. Acupuncture:
   - Studies investigating its potential in reducing itch and improving quality of life in eczema patients
   - Mechanisms still not fully understood

3. Mindfulness and Psychological Interventions:
   - Growing evidence for the role of stress management in eczema care
   - Studies on mindfulness-based stress reduction, cognitive-behavioral therapy, and other psychological interventions

4. Dietary Interventions:
   - Ongoing research into the role of specific nutrients, probiotics, and elimination diets in eczema management
   - Studies on the potential benefits of vitamin D supplementation

5. Natural Products:
  - Investigation of various plant-based compounds for their potential anti-inflammatory and barrier-enhancing properties
  - Focus on understanding mechanisms and ensuring safety and efficacy

While more research is needed, these approaches may offer complementary options for comprehensive eczema management.

Artificial Intelligence and Big Data in Eczema Research

The use of artificial intelligence (AI) and big data analytics is opening new possibilities in eczema research and management:

1. Predictive Modeling:
  - Using AI to predict eczema flares based on various factors (e.g., weather, stress levels, diet)
  - Could potentially allow for more proactive management

2. Image Analysis:
  - AI algorithms for analyzing skin images to assess eczema severity and track treatment progress
  - May improve consistency in eczema assessment and facilitate remote monitoring

3. Personalized Treatment Recommendations:
  - Using machine learning to analyze large datasets and predict which treatments might be most effective for individual patients
  - Could lead to more personalized treatment plans

4. Drug Discovery:
  - AI-driven analysis of molecular data to identify new potential drug targets for eczema
  - May accelerate the drug discovery process

5. Patient-Reported Outcome Analysis:
   - Using natural language processing to analyze patient-reported experiences and identify patterns
   - Could provide valuable insights into the lived experience of eczema and treatment effectiveness

These technological advancements have the potential to revolutionize how we understand, diagnose, and treat eczema.

Challenges in Eczema Research

While the future of eczema treatment looks promising, several challenges remain:

1. Heterogeneity of Eczema:
   - Eczema is not a single condition but a group of related disorders
   - Different subtypes may respond differently to treatments, complicating research

2. Long-Term Safety:
   - Many new treatments lack long-term safety data, particularly important for a chronic condition like eczema

3. Pediatric Considerations:
   - Many new treatments are first tested in adults, leaving gaps in pediatric eczema management
   - Ethical considerations in pediatric clinical trials

4. Cost and Accessibility:
   - Many new treatments, particularly biologics, are expensive
   - Ensuring access to new therapies for all patients who need them is a significant challenge

5. Adherence and Real-World Effectiveness:
  - Translating clinical trial results to real-world effectiveness can be challenging
  - Patient adherence to complex treatment regimens is an ongoing issue

6. Biomarkers and Personalized Medicine:
  - Identifying reliable biomarkers to guide treatment decisions remains a challenge
  - Developing truly personalized treatment approaches is still a work in progress

7. Addressing Comorbidities:
  - Need for treatments that address both eczema and common comorbidities (e.g., asthma, allergies)

8. Prevention:
  - While treatment options are expanding, preventing eczema development remains a significant challenge

Addressing these challenges will be crucial for advancing eczema care and improving outcomes for patients.

The Future of Eczema Care

As research progresses, we can anticipate several trends in the future of eczema management:

1. Precision Medicine:
  - Treatment selection based on individual genetic, immune, and microbiome profiles
  - Tailored approaches that consider the specific subtype and features of a patient's eczema

2. Combination Therapies:
  - Using multiple targeted therapies to address different aspects of eczema pathogenesis
  - Potentially combining topical, systemic, and lifestyle interventions for optimal results

3. Prevention Strategies:
  - Developing interventions to prevent eczema onset in high-risk individuals
  - Focus on early life interventions to modify the course of atopic diseases

4. Holistic Management:
  - Greater integration of physical, psychological, and lifestyle factors in eczema care
  - Emphasis on overall well-being, not just skin symptoms

5. Technology-Enabled Care:
  - Use of digital health tools for monitoring, predicting flares, and guiding treatment
  - Telemedicine and remote monitoring becoming more integral to eczema management

6. Patient Empowerment:
  - Greater involvement of patients in treatment decisions and research priorities
  - Focus on patient-reported outcomes and quality of life measures

7. Addressing Health Disparities:
  - Efforts to ensure new treatments and management strategies are accessible to all patient populations
  - Research into eczema presentation and treatment in diverse skin types and ethnicities

Conclusion: A Bright Future for Eczema Management

The landscape of eczema treatment is evolving rapidly, offering hope for improved management and quality of life for individuals living with this challenging condition. From targeted biologics to microbiome-based therapies, from advanced drug delivery systems to personalized medicine approaches, the future of eczema care looks promising.

Key takeaways:
 - New treatments are targeting specific aspects of eczema pathogenesis with greater precision
 - Personalized medicine approaches are becoming more feasible
 - Technology is playing an increasing role in eczema research and management
 - Holistic approaches that address both skin symptoms and overall well-being are gaining prominence
 - Challenges remain, particularly in terms of long-term safety, cost, and accessibility

For individuals living with eczema, these advancements offer hope for more effective, personalized, and comprehensive care. While not all emerging treatments will prove successful, the breadth and depth of ongoing research suggest that we are entering a new era in eczema management.

As we look to the future, it's important for patients, healthcare providers, and researchers to work together to ensure that new developments translate into real-world benefits for those affected by eczema. By staying informed about emerging treatments and participating in research when possible, individuals with eczema can play an active role in shaping the future of eczema care.

Remember, while we await future breakthroughs, much can be done with current knowledge and treatments. Consistent care, a healthy lifestyle, and a positive outlook remain crucial components of effective eczema management today and in the future.

CHAPTER 14

The Future of Eczema Care: Hope and Empowerment

As we conclude our comprehensive exploration of eczema, it's important to look ahead and consider what the future holds for those living with this challenging condition. In this final chapter, we'll discuss the evolving landscape of eczema care, emphasizing the reasons for hope and the growing empowerment of patients in managing their condition.

Advances in Personalized Medicine

One of the most promising developments in eczema care is the move towards personalized medicine. This approach recognizes that eczema is not a one-size-fits-all condition and that treatment should be tailored to each individual's unique profile.

Key aspects of personalized eczema care:

1. Genetic Profiling:
   - Identifying specific genetic markers associated with different types of eczema
   - Tailoring treatments based on an individual's genetic predisposition

2. Biomarker Analysis:
   - Using blood tests or skin samples to measure specific biomarkers

- Predicting treatment response and disease progression based on these markers

3. Microbiome Mapping:
   - Analyzing an individual's skin microbiome composition
   - Developing targeted treatments to restore microbial balance

4. Immunophenotyping:
   - Detailed analysis of an individual's immune response patterns
   - Selecting immunomodulatory treatments based on specific immune profiles

The promise of personalized medicine lies in its potential to improve treatment efficacy, reduce trial and error in finding effective treatments, and minimize side effects by avoiding unnecessary interventions.

Integrative Approaches to Eczema Management

The future of eczema care is likely to embrace a more holistic, integrative approach that combines conventional medical treatments with complementary therapies and lifestyle modifications.

Components of integrative eczema care:

1. Conventional Treatments:
   - Topical and systemic medications
   - Advanced biologics and targeted therapies

2. Complementary Therapies:
   - Acupuncture
   - Herbal medicine
   - Mind-body techniques (e.g., meditation, yoga)

3. Nutrition and Diet:
  - Personalized dietary plans based on individual triggers and nutritional needs
  - Probiotics and prebiotics for gut and skin health

4. Stress Management:
  - Psychological support and counseling
  - Stress reduction techniques integrated into treatment plans

5. Environmental Modification:
  - Smart home technologies to control environmental triggers
  - Personalized recommendations for clothing, bedding, and skincare products

This integrative approach acknowledges the complex, multifaceted nature of eczema and aims to address all aspects of the condition for comprehensive management.

Technology-Enabled Eczema Care

Advancements in technology are set to revolutionize how eczema is monitored, managed, and treated.

Emerging technologies in eczema care:

1. Wearable Devices:
  - Continuous monitoring of skin parameters (e.g., hydration, pH, temperature)
  - Early detection of flare-ups based on physiological changes

2. Smartphone Apps:
  - Digital symptom tracking and treatment adherence tools
  - AI-powered image analysis for assessing eczema severity

3. Telemedicine:
   - Remote consultations with dermatologists
   - Virtual support groups and education programs

4. 3D-Printed Personalized Skincare:
   - Custom-formulated topical treatments based on individual skin needs
   - On-demand production of personalized emollients and medications

5. Virtual Reality:
   - Distraction therapy for managing itch
   - Immersive patient education experiences

These technological advancements have the potential to improve treatment adherence, facilitate early intervention, and enhance the overall quality of eczema care.

Patient Empowerment and Shared Decision Making

The future of eczema care will likely see a shift towards greater patient empowerment and involvement in treatment decisions.

Key aspects of patient empowerment:

1. Health Literacy:
   - Comprehensive patient education programs
   - Easy access to reliable, up-to-date information about eczema and its treatment

2. Shared Decision Making:
   - Collaborative approach to treatment planning between patients and healthcare providers
   - Tools to help patients understand and weigh treatment options

3. Patient-Reported Outcomes:
   - Greater emphasis on quality of life measures in assessing treatment efficacy
   - Integration of patient-reported data in clinical decision making

4. Self-Management Support:
   - Advanced self-care tools and resources
   - Peer support networks and mentoring programs

5. Patient Advocacy:
   - Increased patient involvement in research priorities and clinical trial design
   - Patient representation in healthcare policy decisions

Empowering patients to take an active role in their care can lead to better treatment adherence, improved outcomes, and greater satisfaction with care.

Addressing Health Disparities in Eczema Care

The future of eczema care must address the significant disparities that exist in access to care and treatment outcomes.

Strategies for reducing disparities:

1. Culturally Competent Care:
   - Training healthcare providers in cultural sensitivity and competence
   - Developing educational materials in multiple languages

2. Improving Access:
   - Telemedicine initiatives to reach underserved communities
   - Community-based eczema care programs

3. Research Inclusivity:

- Ensuring diverse representation in clinical trials
- Studying eczema presentation and treatment efficacy across different ethnicities

4. Addressing Social Determinants of Health:
   - Recognizing and addressing socioeconomic factors that impact eczema care
   - Partnering with community organizations to provide holistic support

5. Policy Advocacy:
   - Pushing for policies that improve access to eczema treatments
   - Advocating for coverage of essential eczema care services by insurance providers

By addressing these disparities, we can work towards a future where effective eczema care is accessible to all, regardless of background or socioeconomic status.

Environmental Sustainability in Eczema Care

As global awareness of environmental issues grows, the future of eczema care will likely place greater emphasis on sustainability.

Sustainable approaches in eczema care:

1. Eco-Friendly Product Formulations:
   - Developing skincare products with biodegradable ingredients
   - Reducing reliance on petrochemicals in eczema treatments

2. Sustainable Packaging:
   - Using recyclable or compostable packaging for eczema products
   - Implementing refill systems to reduce plastic waste

3. Green Pharmacy Practices:
   - Proper disposal methods for unused medications
   - Developing manufacturing processes with lower environmental impact

4. Telemedicine to Reduce Travel:
   - Decreasing the carbon footprint associated with medical visits
   - Utilizing remote monitoring to reduce unnecessary in-person appointments

5. Research into Environmental Triggers:
   - Studying the impact of climate change on eczema prevalence and severity
   - Developing strategies to mitigate environmental risk factors

By considering environmental sustainability in eczema care, we can work towards solutions that are beneficial for both patients and the planet.

The Role of Artificial Intelligence in Eczema Research

Artificial Intelligence (AI) is set to play a significant role in advancing our understanding and treatment of eczema.

Potential applications of AI in eczema care:

1. Drug Discovery:
   - Accelerating the identification of new drug targets
   - Predicting drug efficacy and potential side effects

2. Pattern Recognition:
   - Analyzing large datasets to identify new eczema subtypes
   - Recognizing complex patterns in eczema triggers and progression

3. Predictive Modeling:
   - Forecasting disease progression and treatment outcomes

- Personalizing treatment plans based on individual patient data

4. Image Analysis:
    - Automated assessment of eczema severity from photographs
    - Tracking treatment progress over time

5. Natural Language Processing:
    - Analyzing patient-reported experiences to gain new insights
    - Improving communication between patients and healthcare providers

The integration of AI into eczema research and care has the potential to significantly accelerate progress in the field.

Challenges and Ethical Considerations

While the future of eczema care holds great promise, it also presents several challenges and ethical considerations that must be addressed.

Key challenges and considerations:

1. Data Privacy and Security:
    - Ensuring the protection of sensitive health information
    - Balancing the benefits of data sharing with privacy concerns

2. Equitable Access to Advanced Treatments:
    - Addressing the high costs associated with new therapies
    - Ensuring that advancements benefit all patients, not just those who can afford them

3. Ethical Use of AI and Predictive Technologies:
    - Addressing potential biases in AI algorithms
    - Ensuring transparency in how AI-driven decisions are made

4. Balancing Innovation with Safety:
   - Ensuring rigorous safety testing of new treatments
   - Managing the long-term effects of novel therapies

5. Overdiagnosis and Overtreatment:
   - Avoiding unnecessary interventions as diagnostic capabilities improve
   - Maintaining a balanced approach to eczema management

Addressing these challenges will be crucial in realizing the full potential of future eczema care advancements.

Conclusion: Embracing Hope and Taking Action

As we look to the future of eczema care, there is much reason for hope. Advances in personalized medicine, integrative approaches, technology, and patient empowerment all point towards a future where eczema can be managed more effectively and with greater consideration for individual needs.

However, this bright future is not guaranteed. It will require ongoing effort, research, and advocacy from all stakeholders – patients, healthcare providers, researchers, policymakers, and industry leaders.

For individuals living with eczema, the message is clear: be proactive in your care, stay informed about new developments, and don't hesitate to advocate for yourself and others. The future of eczema care is not just about new treatments and technologies; it's about creating a healthcare ecosystem that truly meets the needs of those living with this challenging condition.

Remember, every step forward in eczema research and care, no matter how small, brings us closer to better management and potentially even prevention or cure. By staying hopeful, engaged, and proactive, we can all contribute to shaping a future where eczema no longer limits quality of life, but is simply another manageable aspect of health.

The journey with eczema may be lifelong, but with ongoing advancements and a commitment to comprehensive, patient-centered care, it's a journey that holds increasing promise for better days ahead. Let this hope inspire action, foster resilience, and drive continued progress in the field of eczema care.

CONCLUSION

Living Well with Eczema - A Holistic Perspective

As we conclude our comprehensive exploration of eczema, it's important to reflect on the key insights we've gained and consider how this knowledge can be applied to improve the lives of those affected by this challenging condition. Eczema is not just a skin disorder; it's a complex, multifaceted condition that impacts every aspect of an individual's life. Throughout this book, we've delved into the science, management strategies, and personal experiences that shape the eczema journey. Now, let's synthesize this information and look ahead to a future of better eczema care and improved quality of life for those living with the condition.

The Evolving Understanding of Eczema

Our journey began with an exploration of what eczema is and how our understanding of it has evolved over time. We've learned that eczema is not a single entity but a group of related conditions characterized by skin inflammation, itching, and a compromised skin barrier. The complexity of eczema's pathophysiology, involving genetic, immunological, and environmental factors, underscores the need for a multifaceted approach to management.

Key takeaways:
  - Eczema is a chronic condition with diverse presentations and triggers

- The interplay between genetics, immune function, and environment is crucial in eczema development
- Understanding the skin barrier's role has revolutionized our approach to eczema care

This evolving understanding has paved the way for more targeted treatments and personalized management strategies, offering hope for better outcomes in the future.

Comprehensive Management Strategies

Throughout this book, we've explored a wide range of management strategies, from conventional medical treatments to lifestyle modifications and alternative therapies. The key message is clear: effective eczema management requires a holistic, individualized approach.

Essential components of eczema management:

1. Skincare routines tailored to individual needs
2. Appropriate use of topical and systemic medications
3. Identification and avoidance of triggers
4. Stress management and psychological support
5. Dietary considerations and nutritional support
6. Environmental modifications
7. Alternative and complementary therapies as appropriate

We've emphasized the importance of working closely with healthcare providers to develop a personalized treatment plan that addresses all aspects of the condition. The goal is not just to manage symptoms but to improve overall quality of life.

The Power of Self-Care and Patient Empowerment

One of the most crucial themes throughout this book has been the importance of self-care and patient empowerment. Living with eczema requires daily attention and care, and those who are most successful in managing their condition are often those who take an active role in their treatment.

Key aspects of patient empowerment:
- Education about eczema and its management
- Development of self-care skills and routines
- Active participation in treatment decisions
- Advocacy for oneself and others with eczema
- Engagement with support networks and resources

By empowering individuals with eczema to take control of their condition, we can improve treatment adherence, outcomes, and overall well-being.

Addressing the Psychological Impact

We've devoted significant attention to the psychological and social aspects of living with eczema, recognizing that the condition's impact extends far beyond the skin. The chronic, visible nature of eczema can affect self-esteem, social relationships, and mental health.

Important considerations:
- The bidirectional relationship between stress and eczema symptoms
- The potential for anxiety and depression in individuals with eczema
- The impact on quality of life, including sleep, work, and social interactions
- The importance of psychological support and coping strategies

By addressing these psychological aspects alongside physical symptoms, we can provide more comprehensive care and support for those living with eczema.

The Role of Lifestyle and Environment

Throughout our exploration, we've highlighted the significant role that lifestyle factors and environmental conditions play in eczema management. From diet and exercise to clothing choices and home environment, many aspects of daily life can influence eczema symptoms.

Key lifestyle considerations:
- Maintaining a balanced, nutrient-rich diet
- Regular, appropriate exercise
- Stress reduction techniques
- Proper sleep hygiene
- Choosing eczema-friendly clothing and bedding
- Creating a skin-friendly home environment

By making informed choices in these areas, individuals with eczema can significantly improve their skin health and overall well-being.

The Promise of Emerging Treatments

Our discussion of current research and emerging treatments has highlighted the exciting developments on the horizon for eczema care. From targeted biologics to microbiome-based therapies, new approaches are offering hope for more effective and personalized treatment options.

Promising areas of research:
- Biologics targeting specific immune pathways
- JAK inhibitors for modulating immune response
- Microbiome-based treatments
- Gene therapy and personalized medicine approaches
- Advanced drug delivery systems

While these developments are promising, it's important to remember that new treatments often take time to become widely available and that their long-term safety and efficacy must be carefully evaluated.

The Importance of Ongoing Research

Throughout this book, we've emphasized the importance of ongoing research in advancing our understanding and treatment of eczema. From basic science investigating the underlying mechanisms of the condition to clinical trials testing new therapies, research is the key to improving outcomes for those with eczema.

Areas requiring further investigation:
  - The complex interplay of genetic and environmental factors in eczema development
    - The role of the microbiome in skin health and eczema
    - Long-term safety and efficacy of new treatments
    - Strategies for preventing eczema development in high-risk individuals
    - The impact of climate change on eczema prevalence and severity

By supporting and participating in eczema research, we can contribute to the advancement of knowledge and the development of better treatments.

Addressing Health Disparities

We've also highlighted the importance of addressing health disparities in eczema care. Factors such as race, ethnicity, socioeconomic status, and geographic location can significantly impact access to care and treatment outcomes.

Key areas for improvement:
    - Increasing diversity in clinical trials
    - Improving cultural competence in healthcare delivery
    - Addressing socioeconomic barriers to care

- Developing educational resources for diverse populations
- Advocating for policies that promote equitable access to eczema treatments

By working to reduce these disparities, we can ensure that advancements in eczema care benefit all individuals, regardless of their background or circumstances.

The Global Perspective

Eczema is a global health concern, and throughout this book, we've tried to maintain an international perspective. While the fundamentals of eczema care are universal, it's important to recognize that factors such as climate, cultural practices, and healthcare systems can influence how eczema is experienced and managed in different parts of the world.

Considerations for global eczema care:
- Adapting management strategies to different climates and environments
- Respecting cultural differences in attitudes towards skin health and treatment
- Addressing challenges in resource-limited settings
- Promoting international collaboration in eczema research and education

By maintaining a global perspective, we can learn from diverse experiences and work towards improving eczema care worldwide.

The Road Ahead: Challenges and Opportunities

As we look to the future of eczema care, we face both challenges and opportunities. The complexity of the condition, the need for personalized approaches, and the ongoing search for more effective treatments all present challenges. However, these challenges also offer opportunities for innovation, collaboration, and improved patient care.

Key challenges and opportunities:
- Developing more targeted and effective treatments
- Improving early diagnosis and intervention
- Enhancing patient education and self-management support
- Leveraging technology for better eczema monitoring and management
- Addressing the economic burden of eczema on individuals and healthcare systems

By facing these challenges head-on and seizing the opportunities they present, we can continue to make progress in eczema care.

A Call to Action

As we conclude this book, it's important to recognize that improving eczema care is a collective responsibility. Whether you're an individual living with eczema, a healthcare provider, a researcher, or a policymaker, there are actions you can take to contribute to better outcomes for those affected by this condition.

For individuals with eczema:
- Stay informed about your condition and treatment options
- Take an active role in your care and treatment decisions
- Practice consistent self-care and adhere to your treatment plan
- Seek support when needed and connect with others who understand your experiences
- Consider participating in eczema research or advocacy efforts

For healthcare providers:
- Stay up-to-date on the latest developments in eczema care
- Take a holistic, patient-centered approach to eczema management
- Address both the physical and psychological aspects of the condition
- Collaborate with other specialists to provide comprehensive care
- Advocate for your patients' needs and access to treatments

For researchers:
- Continue to investigate the underlying mechanisms of eczema
- Pursue innovative approaches to treatment and prevention
- Ensure diversity and inclusivity in clinical trials
- Collaborate across disciplines to advance eczema science
- Engage with patients to understand their experiences and priorities

For policymakers:
- Support funding for eczema research
- Advocate for policies that improve access to eczema care
- Address health disparities in eczema treatment and outcomes
- Promote public awareness and education about eczema

Living Well with Eczema: The Path Forward

As we close this comprehensive exploration of eczema, it's important to remember that despite the challenges this condition presents, it is possible to live well with eczema. With the right knowledge, support, and management strategies, individuals with eczema can lead full, active lives.

The key to living well with eczema lies in:

1. Understanding your condition and its unique manifestations
2. Developing a personalized management plan in partnership with your healthcare providers
3. Practicing consistent self-care and adhering to your treatment regimen
4. Addressing both the physical and emotional aspects of living with eczema
5. Staying informed about new developments in eczema care
6. Connecting with others for support and shared experiences
7. Maintaining hope and a positive outlook, even in challenging times

While eczema may be a lifelong companion for many, it need not define or limit one's life. By embracing a holistic approach to management, leveraging available treatments and support, and maintaining resilience in the face of challenges, those with eczema can thrive.

As we look to the future, there is much reason for hope. Advances in our understanding of eczema, emerging treatments, and a growing emphasis on personalized, patient-centered care all point towards a brighter future for those living with this condition.

Remember, every individual with eczema has a unique journey, but no one needs to walk that path alone. With the knowledge gained from this book, the support of healthcare providers and loved ones, and the strength of the eczema community, we can work together towards a future where eczema is better understood, more effectively managed, and less of a burden on those who live with it.

Let this book serve not as an endpoint, but as a starting point for your journey towards better eczema management and improved quality of life. The road may not always be easy, but with persistence, knowledge, and support, it is possible to find comfort in your skin and joy in your life, eczema notwithstanding.

www.ingramcontent.com/pod-product-compliance
Lightning Source LLC
Chambersburg PA
CBHW070830250726

48662CB00003B/1159